Teaching Nursing

Te

A se

Ch

Pro Vi
Unive
Austra

and

Ru

Nurse
Unive
Austra

CHAPMAN & HALL
London · Weinheim · New York · Tokyo · Melbourne · Madras

Published by
Chapman & Hall, 2–6 Boundary Row, London SE1 8HN, UK

Chapman & Hall, 2–6 Boundary Row, London SE1 8HN, UK

Chapman & Hall GmbH, Pappelallee 3, 69469 Weinheim, Germany

Chapman & Hall USA, 115 Fifth Avenue, New York, NY 10003, USA

Chapman & Hall Japan, ITP-Japan, Kyowa Building, 3F, 2–2–1 Hirakawacho, Chiyoda-ku, Tokyo 102, Japan

Chapman & Hall Australia, 102 Dodds Street, South Melbourne, Victoria 3205, Australia

Chapman & Hall India, R. Seshadri, 32 Second Main Road, CIT East, Madras 600 035, India

First edition 1984

Reprinted 1986, 1989, 1991, 1992, 1994

Second edition 1996

© 1984, 1996 Christine Ewan and Ruth White

This edition is not for sale in North America and Australia; orders from these regions should be referred to Singular Publishing Group, Inc., 4284 41st Street, San Diego, California 92105, USA

Typeset in 10/12pt Palatino by Saxon Graphics Ltd, Derby
Printed in Great Britain by St Edmundsbury Press Ltd, Bury St Edmunds, Suffolk

ISBN 0 412 63280 2

A catalogue record for this book is available from the British Library

∞ Printed on permanent acid-free text paper, manufactured in accordance with ANSI/NISO Z39.48–1992 and ANSI/NISO Z39.48–1984 (Permanence of Paper).

Contents

Preface to the Second Edition

The purpose of this edition is to include the changes in educating nurses following the changes in approaches to teaching and learning in the last decade. With the landmark entry of Nursing as a faculty in the tertiary education sector have come opportunities to reconceptualize nursing education, including the way we think about caring, nursing, teaching and learning. Our original first edition intent remains – that of providing a personal guide for teachers who will use both the new and traditional educational practices as they prepare students to nurse in many health-care arenas in the years beyond this present century.

This edition includes all except one of the original chapters, updated and enlarged. Some have been renamed. Others have been reorganized. There is a new chapter which marks a departure from the first edition in that it addresses education in the workforce, the focus being postgraduates rather than undergraduates. Clinical learning has been given a separate chapter to acknowledge its importance in fostering resolution of the theory–practice debate. The chapter on using learning resources has been omitted. Although it is true that many of the tested and tried learning resources of the classroom described in our first edition retain their usefulness, there are many changes in educational technology. The influence of these changes on the processes of education have yet to be realized and a single chapter in this text would seriously short-change nurse teachers.

The format of self-instructional personal activities and feedback of the first edition has been retained.

We are sure that, like us, nurse educators will note with pleasure the increase in interesting texts written by nurse authors. The new writings of educational theorists have enlarged our view of teaching and learning. We hope we have done justice to them, both in the text and in the list of references.

Christine Ewan
Ruth White
Sydney, December 1995

Introduction to the First Edition

Nursing education is facing a challenging period as the roles of the nurse and the training required to fulfil those roles undergo critical re-examination. This book has been written to provide a personal guide to the new educational practices, and to some of the more traditional approaches, for teachers who will be involved in educating nurses for the future.

The first chapter reviews trends which have emerged in nursing education to equip nurses for their changed roles and responsibilities in the changed environment of modern health services, the second chapter examines the techniques which can be used by teachers or by curriculum planners to determine relevant content for nursing courses and Chapter 3 provides an overview of the learning process presented as the basis for decisions about teaching. Chapter 4 offers guidelines for the choice and design of teaching methods which accommodate both the content and objectives of courses and the learning processes of students. Active student involvement, students' acceptance of responsibility for their own learning, and the development of professional skills and approaches are emphasized. Chapter 5 discusses specific topics in nursing education which require innovative approaches to teaching and learning and provide some examples of applications of the processes and methods discussed in preceding chapters, while the sixth chapter expands on those methods and processes with particular reference to the use of learning resources. Chapter 7 and 8 address the purposes and methods for assessment of student performance and evaluation of courses and teaching. Once again emphasis is placed upon the development among students of professional skills in establishing criteria, using feedback constructively, and evaluating their own and their colleagues' performances.

In keeping with our overall philosophy of the necessity for active involvement of learners in relevant activity, most of the chapters in this book are self-instructional in the sense that they invite the reader to undertake activities which involve analysis of personal teaching conditions and practices, and which encourage the design or development of approaches to specific teaching conditions and problems. Feedback to each of these activities forms the bulk of the text, and it is possible to read the book without undertaking the activities. The decision is yours; however, we recommend the activities to you because they have been chosen from questions most commonly asked by teachers attending our courses and the chances are that many represent questions that you have also asked yourself in the course of your teaching. Attention to the activities will ensure that your personal questions are called to mind and that you are able to apply the content of the feedback to specific aspects of your situation rather than attempting to remember it as general information.

We have attempted to keep the content of the book relatively jargon-free, readable and practical, sometimes at the expense of doing systematic justice to educational theory. We hope that the theorists among our readers will forgive this decision and use the references provided for their specific needs and interests. We also hope that readers with little formal training in educational theory and practice will use this book as an introduction and be stimulated to follow up areas of personal interest among the material offered as references.

Finally, we would wish to acknowledge, with warm appreciation of her skills and gratitude for her unfailing patience, the contribution to this text of Mrs Helen Fodor. The preparation of the manuscript would not have been accomplished without her willing participation in typing, checking and attending to the myriad of details involved.

Trends in nurse education – towards the 21st century

1

INTRODUCTION

What do nurse teachers want to know about teaching nurses in the 21st century? What will be so different? It is necessary only to point to the awesome advances in medical science, technology, electronic communication or to the political, economic or social movements influencing the values, lifestyles and health behaviours of populations, to conclude that preparing health professionals, including nurses, is a formidable task **now**, in the 1990s. So what is the challenge?

It seems that the challenge is the rate of change itself. The next 20 years will experience a greater rate of change than any previous 20-year period in history (Ball *et al.*, 1988). The question for this text is, of course, how will nurse education be affected? Certainly there are many changes in the way we view learning and teaching and a continual review of new approaches is an important component of the work of curriculum developers, and classroom and clinical teachers. There can be little argument that awareness of national or of world forces leads us to think through the relevance of what is taught to students and to consider the context in which students will practise on graduation.

Our task in this introductory chapter is, therefore, to outline some of the trends in nurse education in considering how to help students to learn, how to assist graduate students and professionals to learn in the workplace, and how to recognize the values and ethical issues which are gaining in importance as technology and biomedical science increasingly demand difficult decisions.

CHANGES AND CHALLENGES

Within nurse education itself movements (such as professionalization, specialization) have exerted their impact and demanded a response in the past. In the 1990s the pattern of response is largely influenced by the increasing numbers of nurses with postgraduate degrees. The analysis of professional issues and the investigation into questions of education, administration and clinical practice has increased. In turn, the 21st century is likely to be a thriving era for research into nursing practice. Notwithstanding the changes taking place in the women's movement in the present decade, its effect on raising awareness of the general population (and nurses in particular) of the legitimacy of human rights in a broad sense and patient's rights in the context of health and welfare has not diminished. Furthermore, the increasing numbers of women seeking endorsement for political office could be a significant future influence, particularly regarding issues such as the redistribution of social resources in the community (see Sawer and Sims, 1993).

Several issues stand out as being significant for nurse education:

- knowledge and knowledge production;
- technology and education;
- specialization;
- professionalization;
- political and economic issues;
- social and cultural issues.

KNOWLEDGE AND KNOWLEDGE PRODUCTION

In the 1980s, 'knowledge explosion' was a household word popularized by Toffler (1981) with his picture of an information bomb exploding in our midst. Now the effect of that explosion on the acceleration of change is described by Toffler and Toffler (1993, p 247) not as a metaphorical bomb but an actual arsenal in waiting. 'This acceleration, partly driven by faster communication, means that hot-spots can materialize and war erupt into the global system almost overnight. Dramatic events demand response before governments have had time to digest their significance. Politicians are forced to make more and more decisions about things they know less and less about at a faster and faster rate.' Responses to global emergencies require health professionals, nurses among them, to have special skills. Could their preparation ever be sufficient for meeting the needs of these enormous human tragedies?

Beare and Slaughter (1993) point to a new paradigm made up of a synthesis of three major shifts in our approach to knowledge production:

- superseding the industrial materialist framework;

- superseding the false duality about human beings and their environment;
- superseding scientific materialism.

The authors claim that such a new paradigm provides 'a new and wider framework, one which includes science but which saves us from being bluffed by a part pretending to be the whole. It opens up dimensions of human experience which are the most ennobling and transcendent' (p 71). Certainly such a focus puts new life into education and presents educational planners with a different set of constructs as a basis for designing individual as well as state and national programmes.

It is now possible not only to marvel at the explanations of phenomena but to experience humankind's advances by, for example, walking in space, retrieving vast displays of information, 'seeing' inside the human body at fractional depths and angles through integrated computerized imaging. We can now contemplate 'new forms of "learning" via chemical or electronic implants, inter-species communication, genetic counselling and many other shifts, social innovations and new types of technology (including nuclear fusion, expert systems and space manufacturing). The combined effects of such changes are powerful, bewildering, and essentially unpredictable' (Beare and Slaughter, 1993, p 8). One effect is, however, obvious. Education for specialists in a rapidly changing world will challenge educational planners, while education for multiskilled generalists will continue to be in demand.

TECHNOLOGY, HEALTH AND EDUCATION

Technology is changing the way we live. 'Nanotechnology' (tiny machines fabricating sophisticated materials) is predicted 'to overturn economic systems, transform the natural and built environments, revolutionize health care, defence and space travel' (Beare and Slaughter, 1993, p 6). Scarcely a sphere of society, let alone education, has been unaffected by the advances in technology. The tools of education now include individual tutorials by computer, mixed media CD ROM and small- and large-group teaching by teleconferencing. The organization of programmes is no longer constrained by size of class or presence of teacher since mass communication by satellite is a reality.

The information superhighway is a household word. The ease with which children have access to and manage video and computer games has a direct impact on our ideas of how students learn. Now that it is possible to link numbers of institutions to access results from various research studies and to store, analyse and retrieve data, the implications for educational research have yet to be realized. Exploiting the new technologies for education, industry and the professions is a required skill for educational planners and teachers.

Sophisticated technology has been increasing its impact on the health-care system, not only in the availability of a range of diagnostic tests but, also, in increasing the safety, validity and reliability of test results. The variety of therapies at the disposal of health professionals has increased. The implications of the new technologies are as wide-ranging for medical and health-services research as they are for education, producing on the one hand, hope for previously untreatable conditions and on the other, complex problems for ethical decision-makers forced to choose among many needy individuals for the limited and astronomically expensive technological resources.

Beare and Slaughter (1993, p 166) address the question in relation to education for the 21st century:

> It is our observation that when low-level human motives such as fear, greed, and hostility become associated with powerful technologies, the result is indeed a long-running disaster. (. . .) But when higher motives such as selfless love, stewardship and what Buddhists call 'loving kindness' come into play, there are interesting consequences. (. . .) When a right relationship is re-established between people, culture and technology, a new world of options emerges.

Penzias, in 1989, after investigating issues of managing in a high-tech world, believes that only an integrated sharing of information can bring benefits to human society. 'As I see it, we need an integrated approach to quality, one that defines and realizes the performance of each system in its entirety, rather than the small-scale behaviour of its pieceparts. Technology that is measured by its total impact on the human beings it serves provides a worthy goal for the information age' (p 199).

THE SPECIALIZATION ISSUE

The diversity in educational courses in specialties is, of course, a response to the increase in knowledge and technology and the resulting specialization in specific areas of knowledge, expertise or technique. As a driving force in health care, specialization has splintered broad areas of treatment into smaller specialties and the rate of technological change has involved the specialist in an endless study and pursuit of the most up-to-date advances.

Nursing is not immune to this pressure. At discussions of the International Council of Nursing (ICN), the growing movement of post-basic specializations and regulation of its development was a matter of growing concern. The concern is that specialties at post-basic level offered at universities would, in time, be defined by university course titles. As there is a plethora of titles across states and among different countries, it is difficult to see how the goals of international nursing, of consistency, parity and unity, would be met (Parkes, 1994).

The increasing numbers of nurses enrolling in Faculties of Education at graduate level has had an interesting effect on staff members whose expertise is in primary and secondary schooling and general education at university level. Enter a new specialty – nursing education – with clinical education as its urgent need. 'Very few staff have direct experience of teaching and learning in these other institutional contexts' (Crittenden, 1994). Undoubtedly, change is not all one way; nursing education is affected by its context in university education, but clearly, university education is being changed by the presence of nurse education and highly qualified nurse graduates.

PROFESSIONALIZATION

Swayed by issues of the status of the expert, the power of superior knowledge and technology, and the rewards that accompany specialist expertise, professionalization has been a powerful force for some time, affecting most of the labour force. Education and health care have not escaped and nurse education has a history of progressive rise on the professional ladder. A criticism often made of a profession aiming for recognition of its role in society *vis-à-vis* the service it provides, is the issue of status-seeking. Furthermore, attempts to improve the education foundation of a profession and the qualification of its members are often labelled with the accusation of credentialism.

Not surprisingly, powerful forces challenge both the legitimacy of the expert and the status of professional eminence. Human rights, conservation, self-help, community action, alternative education and health movements, and 'clean up the world' groups, for example, are vocal, visible and attract an influential following. The result is that, increasingly, professionals, including nurses, have to prove their worth in society.

POLITICAL AND ECONOMICAL ISSUES

The macro-structure in which nursing education is planned is subject to political decisions about its future expansion or contraction, economic strictures on the provision of resources and materials and the social responsibility to take a stand on many world issues such as nuclear involvement, removal of land mines, population control or the environment.

In the western world there are forces impinging upon nursing education arising directly out of the health-care system itself. For example, the contentious arguments about the advantages and disadvantages of high technology, the claim that redress of balance between acute and preventive care is overdue, and the often painful decisions required in bioethics, are areas of concern indicating the complexities in modern health care.

It would be hard to find a country whose health system was not affected by current political and economic forces. Day surgery is set to increase to about 60% of hospital surgery by the year 2000. Aftercare in the client's own home will also increase, changing the distribution of personnel and resources.

'Advances in medical research are making possible more and more interventions every year to treat the diseases of the very elderly. Those people – indeed everyone over 65 years of age – have health needs that are colossal, constantly increasing and, theoretically, given the march of science, infinitely expandable' (Konner, 1993, p 144). The implications for decision-making on the distribution of resources among the health care of other groups, as well as the aged, such as families with children or the education of the young, concern politicians, ethicists as well as health-care professionals.

The developing world's concern with day-to-day demands for the essentials of food, water, shelter and safety put the previous problems into a perspective often unappreciable by many who will use this book. North–south comparisons between the resources spent on research into heart disease and other 'western lifestyle' diseases, and that spent on such widespread diseases as cholera or malaria or HIV/AIDS in the developing world, reveal scant ability to progress on a world-health scale.

SOCIAL AND CULTURAL FORCES

Few would not agree that stress-related factors in modern societies are increasing. Biological stress from threatened disease or chronic illness, social stress from an often self-inflicted heavy work and life schedule, emotional and psychological stress from fear, abuse, alienation or the pain of unemployment and homelessness, present cycles of stressful living that are all too common. Scattered rural communities as well as large urban complexes are affected.

Stress-reduction techniques using community education, warning against depending on minor tranquillizers, the use of community resources, activities and programmes emphasizing exercise, relaxation and encouraging lifestyle and environmental changes may be effective in encouraging individuals to implement stress reduction. Where the individual is powerless to effect change, forces such as lobby groups to influence government decisions on the environment, housing, work safety and employment assume importance for health professionals in attempting to reduce the effects of social and behavioural illness (Riddell and Wright, 1991).

RESPONSES TO THE CHANGES AND CHALLENGES

Recent writers in nursing know about the challenges. The articles and books talk of 'reform of nurse education', 'curriculum revolution' and 'reconceptualizing clinical education'. The challenges are not seen as oppressive but as mainsprings of action, spurs to find different solutions and the stimulus needed to spark new ideas. The writing is refreshing, devastatingly honest and sceptical. Recent examples, among many, are Lawler's (1991) article 'In search of an Australian identity', Lumby's (1995) article 'Researching the knowing through the knower', and the text by Lathlean and Vaughan (1994), *Unifying Nursing Practice and Theory*.

There is also writing that is courageous in pursuing ideas, topics and concepts in depth while at the same time revealing personal journeys and attempts at bringing about change. Again, many examples could be quoted; among them are Reed and Procter's (1993) text, *Nurse Education: A Reflective Approach*, Andersen's (1991) article 'Mapping the terrain of the discipline' and Emden's (1991) personal journey, 'Ways of knowing in nursing'.

New captions have appeared as a shorthand way of indicating the focus of some of the recent developments: 'the knowledgeable doer' (Perry and Jolley, 1991), 'the reflective practitioner' (originally described by Schon, 1983, but now used as currency by many researchers, curriculum specialists and educators and clinicians) and 'advanced practitioners' (Reed and Procter, 1993).

If we add to these works the advances in the skills of the clinical specialists and clinical nurses, who are increasingly respected for their clinical and practical knowledge, the future for teaching and learning in the classroom, clinical setting and workplace looks positive indeed.

TECHNOLOGY AND NURSING

It is no longer surprising to see the use of intelligent robotics in industry performing delicate procedures once performed by human technicians. Their introduction into other sectors of society cannot be far behind. How realistic is the use of robotics in health care? Some of the imaginative devices portrayed in films may not be too far removed from daily life, for example, 'technologically based wristwatches, providing continuous monitoring of our physical status and perhaps even ... drug dispensing capabilities automatically triggered by our physiological and biochemical needs' (Ball *et al.*, 1988, p 9). If so, the authors ask, will the judgement of nurses be secondary to the rules incorporated in equipment if thoughtful technical and clinical work is automated?

Cox, Harsanyi and Dean (1987, p 5) quote from Schwirian (1983, p 1) that the 'computer revolution will change nursing practice in the next 20 years more than nursing has changed in the past century'.

Teaching and learning will also change through the computer revolution. O'Brien and Walton (1993) describe an information retrieval and analysis package for students in learning to access and critically appraise information sources.

Practitioners and teachers are becoming more aware of computer-assisted learning, and are applying the psychological and physiological principles of ergonomics in their use of personal computers and also in the application of those principles to nursing care. Problem-based, patient-related learning strategies are being developed by videodisc; microcomputer and voice recognition are being incorporated into clinical simulations for education in the health professions (Ball *et al.*, 1988).

By the year 2000 nurses must be capable of understanding and working in health care which will be driven by increasingly sophisticated technology. This will include, to a greater extent than previously, caring for people who are victims of the effects of a technological society – the alienated, the unemployed and those who feel devalued and shut out of the productive sections of society.

At the other end of the spectrum, the spiralling costs associated with the production and employment of technology points to the need for education in the design of low-cost 'appropriate technology'. The dilemma that exists in the 'throw-away' society is a fine point between protection from infection and the fair distribution of resources to society as a whole.

An important trend influencing the care of children, particularly, in developing countries, is the application of appropriate technology to solve problems on a community as well as on an individual scale. The simple method of administration of oral rehydration has demonstrated the dramatic curative effect of timely, low-cost, highly relevant, easily prepared and administered technology. Nurse educators have an important role to play in indicating the importance of 'low' technology, as well as the visible 'high' technology.

Preparing nurses for practice in the age of information requires an education to maintain relevancy in a rapidly changing technological environment, to use personal and therapeutic skills of 'touch' to communicate with unconscious patients, and to apply technical, co-ordinating and monitoring skills.

The accelerated trend for nursing education to include ethical decision-making in the nursing programme is directly related to the dilemmas raised by technological change. Levine (1988) reminds us of the potential of machines to depersonalize nurses and patients, and the need to protect each other from the indifference of the machine.

EMPOWERING PRACTITIONERS

The World Health Organization's concept of empowerment for nurses came from the announcement of the Director General, Halfdan Mahler. Unleashing a powerhouse for change and 'empowering nurses in order to empower the people they serve' became the catchcry of the early 1980s (Clay, 1992). As a response to the political and economic forces responsible for the distribution of wealth and resources, primary health care is a powerful trend towards integration of services in the interests of the provision of basic human needs. For nurse education, the trend is important as it is necessary to prepare nurses to discover different lifestyles and different communities. Educational programmes in nursing with a strong hospital orientation require review to widen the experiences of students. Bringing people into decision-making requires skills which need to be fostered through practice. For the student who learns that nursing is predominantly a one-to-one relationship, dealing with community groups may be outside 'nursing'. Primary health care involves the nurse in actively assisting people and groups in self-determination and in making decisions based on their own goals.

Primary health care is also a response to the social and cultural forces impinging on the rights of individuals. Health personnel no longer hold the monopoly of knowledge. In fact, unless the community assists the professional to understand what primary health care means in their particular context, a barrier between them will exist and knowledge will not be shared.

In the primary health-care approach, care actions cannot be dissociated from social actions, since everything that affects health has a social element. This means re-emphasizing the social dimension of nursing and recognizing its social influence as well as the link with other networks of health and social action.

TOWARDS A DISCIPLINE OF NURSING

The recognition of nursing as a discipline involves 'a unique perspective, a distinct way of viewing all phenomena, which ultimately defines the limits and nature of its inquiry' (Donaldson and Crowley, 1978). In the years since Donaldson and Crowley's perspective the work on evolving the discipline has accelerated. Andersen (1991) counsels that the process of discipline exploration has some long way to go. Most of the writers in Gray and Pratt (1991) *Towards a Discipline of Nursing*, attest to the influence of the entry of nursing into the tertiary education sector in intensifying the urge to develop nursing as an academic study with its full knowledge base.

A debating point is the issue of scientific problem-solving as the preferred mode for nursing practice. Those who support this view do so from the conviction that problems form the basis of practice and that following the steps of problem-solving is a rational, respected scientific method. Those who find this stance unsatisfactory do so from two main standpoints. One holds that intuition should not be discounted as a nursing skill and that intuitive reasoning should not be devalued and omitted from nursing practice. The other claims that a limited view of problem-solving obtains when computerized programmes break down the components of a person's problem into small bits. At that point, appreciation of the whole person is almost a lost perspective. The trend to analyse critically the divergent view expressed in nursing is a healthy sign of colleagueship and security in the ability to admit a different view.

Faced with the growing pressure to identify 'what is nursing', the trend in many countries is to claim that the whole person is the focus of nursing. That both 'whole' and 'health' derive from the same root, *hal*, is confirmation for many nurses that the whole person and health are valid concepts strengthening each other, providing a rationale for the current concern about health as well as illness.

Some nurses believe that what is distinctive about nursing, therefore, is that nurses take their priorities directly from the patient/client (whole person) rather than from the treatment regime, the disease process or the technological prescription. This puts an emphasis on phenomena that have always claimed the attention of nurses during their span of contact with patients, which, until recently, have not been studied nor investigated for their importance in patient comfort, care or cure. Examples of these phenomena are emergence of pain, restlessness, discomfort and dependence.

Teachers are often in a dilemma when confronted with the question of whether to teach for current practice or whether to make students more aware of the trends in nursing knowledge with which they will have to deal later as graduates. The issue seems to be whether teachers consider nursing as a subject worthy of serious study and scholarship, an emerging discipline in its own right, or a field of professional practice, or both of these.

The issue of relevance of the curriculum to current practice is important, but equally important is the option of assisting students to think towards the future, extending their ideas about human welfare and their own potential for effectiveness in health care. In a world of such rapid change as we are experiencing, the 'need for preparation for change' is a cliché – overused and out of date. A future orientation seems unarguable. Moreover, there are many sources of assistance available now to nurse teachers seeking to revitalize their teaching or to study curriculum development. A growing literature and the existence of professional groups interested in educational development both within nursing and across the disciplines is evidence of increasing activity in the field of health professional education generally and nurse education in particular.

SUMMARY

What do Virginia Henderson and Ivan Illich have in common? It is not just that their famous early writings became required reading in nursing and medical schools. Well-thumbed copies of *The Nature of Nursing* (Henderson, 1966) and *Medical Nemesis* (Illich, 1976) can be found on most nurse educators' desks or not too far away on their office shelves. Not only because these authors shook a few foundations in their day, important as that has been. What they have in common in this latter day is that both have written re-affirmations of what they wrote 25 years or so ago.

Illich says: 'After a quarter of a century, I am still satisfied with the substance and rhetoric of *Nemesis*' (Illich, 1995), and Henderson's sentiment is similar, that after 25 years the statement still reflects her concept of the nature of nursing (Henderson, 1991). Both acknowledge the immense changes in the world of health care, yet both are not susceptible to fashions but retain the values of their observations of the 60s and 70s.

Reading the statements of these two luminaries in the health-care world is a salutary experience. We are so influenced by the awesome changes around us, in science, medicine, technology and electronics, that our natural tendency is to expect that we must respond to the changes with 'new' and appropriate alternatives to our 'old' ways.

What does this tell us about writing a second edition of a text like *Teaching Nursing*? In the first edition we examined the forces impinging on nurse education and then suggested the responses that nursing and nurse education were making, or should be making, to each one. While it is not argued that the context of health care and nurse education remains uninfluenced by change, in this second edition we have been far more cautious in suggesting how nursing education should change to reflect the future demands. Rather, we have acknowledged that the values which attracted nurse educators into teaching and learning in the first place are still appropriate and need to be preserved as the 21st century approaches.

Deciding what to teach 2

INTRODUCTION

While deciding how to teach is as important as (some would say more important than) deciding what to teach, choices from the vast amount of content available are inevitable. Brookfield (1991, p 22) claims that 'being clear about what you teach is crucial but it is not enough in and of itself; you must be able to communicate to your students the values, beliefs, and purposes comprising your rationale'.

Whatever your role in teaching students to nurse you will have some responsibility in deciding what you will teach, and you will have a rationale for the choices you make. Even though you may be given a prescribed area or topic with little room to manoeuvre, the emphasis you choose to give to components of the topic will quickly indicate to students your preferences, values and goals.

The purpose of this chapter is to identify ways of determining relevant content for teaching nursing. Relevant for what and for whom are issues that will be threaded through the activities and discussion as they are basic to the decisions teachers make in choosing content.

Although it is true that deciding what to teach is largely a question for the total curriculum, it is not the intention in this text to discuss curriculum design and structure in detail. There are several informative texts on curriculum planning in nurse education (e.g. Conley, 1973; Torres and Stanton, 1982; Jolley and Allan, 1986; Greaves, 1987; Bevis and Watson, 1989; Bevis, 1982; Quinn, 1994) and many in general education (e.g. Taba, 1962; Warwick, 1973; Stenhouse, 1975; Kerr, 1976; Skilbeck, 1984; Smith and Lovat, 1990; Brady, 1992) where curriculum issues may be read in detail. On the other hand there are few resources to assist the teacher in classroom, clinical or community teaching (be they trained teachers or clinicians who teach only occasionally) to decide what should be taught in relation to a particular group or class of students in the context of health services.

In using the format of activities, feedback and discussion, it is hoped that day-to-day issues and problems in selecting relevant teaching material will surface and that the suggested techniques for choosing content will prove useful.

When you finish this chapter you should be able to recognize the basis of the decision you take in choosing what to teach and be able to use a variety of techniques for determining content in assisting students to learn to nurse.

WHY IS DECIDING WHAT TO TEACH SUCH A PROBLEM IN NURSING?

There are educators and writers in general education who believe that some content can be learned for its own sake; that it has intrinsic value. 'Training the mind' is often the justification. In the health professions where licensure for practice follows a course, the view is that content has value only if it is useful. For example, in medical education Cox claims that 'knowledge which cannot be used is useless' (Cox, 1987). The debates continue and within them the justification for elective studies in general education subjects in nursing courses is often argued on the premise that a broad education is desirable in professional practitioners.

When we consider that 'few subjects have "static" or unchanging content' (Brady, 1992) and that nursing content is directly influenced by changes in technology, medicine and science, the problem for nurse educators is a major one. Add to that the proposition offered by social and political scientists that 'if nurses are able to understand the competing forces which help to shape them and the nature of their work (. . .) they can help to produce their times by participating in the important struggles of the day in a socially and politically informed manner' (Kenway and Watkins, 1994, p 2). Selecting what to teach appears to be a critical decision. How can the decision be made?

APPROACHES TO COURSE CONTENT

ACTIVITY

Choose an area or topic you are currently teaching, or planning to teach, and make a list of what you consider your students must know. In your list underline the most important items. Find a colleague and explain your rationale, justifying your selection of 'most important' items.

FEEDBACK

Naturally enough you may have found this activity irritating, as it is such a fundamental question to answer and obviously there are no right or wrong answers. In explaining your rationale you may have found a few contentious issues. The point of the activity is, of course, the task of identifying the basis of your decisions about what to teach.

USING A CURRICULUM MODEL

Imagine that your faculty have recently completed the initial stages of curriculum development and have arrived at consensus on the choice of a curriculum model, which has been chosen for its suitability to direct the selection of essential areas of content. For example Beddome *et al.* (1995) report a curriculum philosophy developed by faculty members and informed by 'feminist, humanistic, existential, phenomenological and socially critical orientations'. The faculty emphasized clinical experience as a central focus for the curriculum. This resulted in a Delphi survey of practising nurses in the four regions to be served by the curriculum to discover what the nurses of the future will need to **do**, **know** and **be** to provide high-quality nursing care. The results in order of priority were:

1. Have increased accountability and responsibility for their practice
2. Make decisions
3. Liaise with other disciplines and agencies
4. Think critically
5. Teach the public
6. Use community resources
7. Do more assessments
8. Act as change agent
9. Leadership
10. Perform nursing functions autonomously.

The authors emphasized the value of collaboration between educators and practitioners in the development of a new curriculum for the 21st century. The inclusion of experienced practitioners in decisions about what to teach seems an obvious choice. In addition, surveys of recent graduates are also valuable as their experience of their education, both theoretical and practical, and their reactions to it, are likely to be strong and pertinent. Your school may have the results of such surveys. It is a good idea to make use of this material to assist in your decisions about content and how it is taught. However, some of the illusions we hold about teaching nursing can be shattered by listening to what students regard as 'nursing'. Melia (1982) found that students' descriptions of nursing can be summed up in three ways:

- real nursing, i.e. technically oriented work;
- not really nursing, i.e. social care, such as long-stay geriatric patients;
- just basic nursing, i.e. nursing care which is independent of medical prescription.

Since Melia's study the advances in technology, science and medicine are awesome and the resulting changes in specialization in nursing continue to draw stark comparisons between so called 'high-visibility' and 'low-visibility' nursing. One view suggests that health care is moving towards 'a skill construction which has as its basis a view of knowledge which is technical and "scientific"' (Kenway and Watkins, 1994). On the other hand, it is good to realize that in nursing the challenge has been recognized and there is an emphasis on the importance of constructing nursing knowledge out of nursing practice (Lumby, 1995).

Whatever the curriculum model your school uses its central focus will provide you with guidelines from which you can determine the content for your course.

APPLYING CLINICAL RESEARCH FINDINGS AND 'LEARNING FROM EXPERIENCE'

Lindeman (1989) points to the two distinct meanings of clinical practice. One is the application of existing knowledge, the other is the knowledge that comes from the experience itself. It is the latter knowledge that Tanner (1988) claims should form a significant component of the content learned in the classroom. Tanner claims that we do not need more formal models but rather that classroom learning needs to be 'the application of practice rather than the other way around' (p 214). Lindeman (1989, p 24) states that 'clinical learning should build knowledge not just use it'.

The 'curriculum revolution' literature is replete with renewed emphases on the preparation of graduates who can function well in a rapidly changing health-care environment. The result of a Delphi survey to identify priorities in research in nurse education placed as the no. 1 priority 'integration of research findings into nursing curriculum' (Tanner and Lindeman, 1987).

MacLeod and Farrell (1994) report on a 'practice-driven approach to curriculum' in a Canadian initiative and point to the importance of experience and the relevance of practical knowledge. Students and practitioners worked together. The approach described notes that it is 'practice-driven and phenomenological'. Nursing care, research, education and administration are in continuous interaction, each building on and nourishing the others.

Reflective processes in learning and practice have gained in popularity since Schon's *The Reflective Practitioner* (1983) and *Educating the Reflective Practitioner* (1988) interpreted Dewey's (1938) *Experience and Education* in the light of current-day professional practice and teaching. Holloway and Race note the interest of professional nursing in a reflective and reflexive practitioner who can exercise autonomy for decision-making. These qualities and skills are important in the context of increased managerial control apparent in some organizations (Holloway and Race, 1993).

Your school may be dissatisfied with a traditional behaviourist approach and, like Lindeman (1989), have found that 'patients and clinical situations do not match the nice neat boxes associated with the traditional approach'. This does not mean that traditional subjects will be discarded but that the central focus is on the content that underpins clinical and professional practice. This is supported in the United Kingdom, as documented in the Department of Health (Nursing Division) publication *A Strategy for Nursing* (1989 – quoted in Perry and Jolley, 1991): 'All clinical practice should be founded on up-to-date information and research findings; practitioners should be encouraged to identify the needs and opportunities for research presented by their work'.

USING COMPETENCIES

The programme in which you teach may have accepted the competency approach where all of the competencies necessary for practice as a professional nurse have been determined, as well as a system of evaluation. Labunski (1991) describes a programme of competencies designed to achieve standardization but also to guide the selection of content. Given that it is well known that students will learn most efficiently that which is examinable, it is likely that your teaching will be directed mainly toward ensuring that the competencies are fully covered. As you peruse the competencies you may, of course, wish to expand specific areas and particularly embed them in a context which gives students a well rounded education.

The Australian Nursing Council Incorporated (ANCI) competencies have been designed to provide the registering authorities in each state in Australia with a set of 'nationally agreed minimum competencies that would be acceptable to all of the nurse registering authorities for the initial registration and enrolment of nurses' (Australian Nursing Council, 1994). Although not designed as a resource for curriculum development, the detailed statements of domains, competencies, verbal descriptions and cues give a specific guide to what needs to be learned and what standard of performance students should strive to achieve.

The competency movement is not without its critics as well as its supporters. While it is true that the technical education sector has accepted competencies, in general, the university sector to date has not. Social critics foresee the competency movement playing into the hands of government control and claim 'it is useful to consider the part that competencies credentials play in the cultural struggle for prestige and power' (Kenway and Watkins, 1994, p 28).

Support for competencies (apart from nurses themselves) comes from one part of the university sector (Jackson, 1995). Certainly not at the level of detail of Labunski (1991) or the Australian Nursing Council (1994), but the concept of competencies is similar. In Jackson's opinion the idea of competencies has been mistakenly dismissed in universities as being suitable only to vocational training. 'The concept is elastic enough to include the highest cognitive development that can be achieved in the best university education.' The seven competencies Jackson identifies are:

- access to existing knowledge;
- command of existing knowledge;
- criticism of existing knowledge;
- exploration of issues with existing knowledge;
- creation of new knowledge;
- identification of ethical dimensions of a problem or issue;
- teamwork with peers to achieve objectives.

These competencies, with the addition of critical and emancipatory skills, are similar to those recommended by Carr and Kemmis (1986) as attributes of critical professional performance. Jackson adds that any discipline would have its own special competencies (Jackson, 1995).

Remember, we are focusing on deciding what to teach, so what is the justification for the decision a nursing faculty might take to use competencies as the basis of their choice of content? Gonczi, Haager and Oliver (1990) explain that competency-based standards show clearly what a person has to be able to do in order to demonstrate that she/he can practise successfully as a professional.

PREPARING THE KNOWLEDGEABLE DOER

Hogston (1993) found in nursing literature that competence is commonly believed to 'incorporate values, critical thinking, clinical judgement , formulation of attitudes and integration of practice and theory'. He adds that being competent is much more than the application of knowledge and skill and points to the skills of analysis and synthesis of clinical judgement. Furthermore, these are essential for the 'knowledgeable doer'. His views are supported by Perry and Jolley (1991), Reed and Procter (1993), Lumby (1995) and many more who agree that nursing is more than doing, because thinking and doing interact in nursing practice, making nurses more than technicians.

APPLYING EDUCATIONAL CRITERIA

Brady (1992) gives a commonly cited criterion list for determining curriculum content and cautions that the criteria should be applied to all suggested content to be taught in a course and not applied in isolation. He cites the following criteria:

- **validity**: whether the content is authentic and whether it can achieve stated objectives;
- **significance**: whether the content is fundamental to the subject or field in question; whether the content selected allows for breadth and depth of treatment;
- **interest**: whether the content is of interest to students;
- **learnability**: whether the content is easily learnable;
- **consistency with social realities**: whether the content represents the most useful orientation to the world;
- **utility**: whether the content is useful to the student in coping with his or her life.

Let's summarize the approaches we have discussed so far which influence the decisions about content:

- using a curriculum model;
- applying research findings and 'learning from experience';
- using competencies for safe, professional nursing care;
- preparing knowledgeable doers, combining thinking and doing;
- applying educational criteria.

CRITERIA FOR CONTENT SELECTION

It is important to be aware of the variety of ways that content can be selected, the justifications given for each approach, the supporting arguments and the critical evaluations made. Your course might include strands of all the approaches mentioned above as well as others more appropriate to your general or specialty area. Clearly, there are many ways to design a course. The decisions are rarely taken by one person, but usually by the faculty who will be involved. However, in your class, with your students, you are faced with decisions about what students will learn and, importantly, how they will learn. This situation introduces learning principles that determine the priorities you give to the method of presentation to students, their participation and their expectations that what they are learning translates into practice.

ACTIVITY

Imagine you are fortunate enough to have a long lead-time to prepare to teach your course. Also, you have been given a free hand to select the content. As you survey the increases in scientific knowledge, the complexities of modern health services and your particular group of students, what criteria will you have in mind to help you to select the content of your course from the many valid options?

FEEDBACK

The first criterion is an obvious one. Because nursing is a practical profession what is taught must be relevant to practice. Practical knowledge gained through experience and brought into the classroom exemplifies the kind of relevance championed by Tanner and Lindeman (1987). Bevis and Watson (1989) note that relevance, reality and practice are the key to determining content 'so that not only does theory inform practice, but practice informs theory'.

Second, because the content chosen will be the focus of student learning, it should be consistent with the way students will learn subject matter, learn how to translate it into practice and learn how to nurse.

Learning and the learner make up the third criterion. This criterion may not be so obvious but in recent years the number of nurses who are prepared to present their values and beliefs about nursing, man, health or community, to name only a few elements, is increasing. The criterion for choosing content, for them, is the perspective they hold on what nursing is, and about how nursing should be practised, taught and researched.

It may be interesting at this stage to compare the above criteria with those advocated by Brady (1992) cited above. You may have listed additional criteria such as the time available, accessibility of resources or type of facilities for teaching. The latter may include whether you will teach mainly in the classroom or in a practical setting in a hospital, or a community. Those aspects are certainly important as they can facilitate your planning or be a major constraint on what is possible to include in a course. Some of these aspects are dealt with in other chapters. In this chapter we will concentrate more on the criteria that you as a teacher personally choose in deciding what your students will learn.

RELEVANCE

There is a full discussion in the next chapter on relevance as one of the conditions for learning. Its importance for motivating students and for making learning meaningful is argued. In this chapter our concern is more with relevance as a criterion for the selection of what to teach in the first place. Logically, decisions about content lead to the organization of learning sessions to enable students to appreciate the relevance of what they are learning to the accomplishment of a personal or professional goal.

If you have ever had the misfortune of being locked into a course where the teacher's choice of content was really meant for some other group of students, or was chosen because of a personal preference – or bias – but had no link with its translation into practice, you will have experienced a very interesting and possibly expert course of lectures, but you will have been left wondering about your ability to perform competently as a result of your experience.

The focus on relevance in deciding content in this text relates to the needs of students, which are influenced by:

- their prior knowledge of the subject;
- their background and experience;
- their aspirations and the context in which they hope to realize them;
- the activities (professional nursing acts) they will have to perform as graduates in current practice;
- their perception of future tasks and activities in changing health services;
- the roles they will enact in the performance of those activities;
- the context in which they will function.

A criticism often made of this approach is that patients and their needs and problems rather than students' needs should be the primary focus of decisions about content of nursing courses. However, while such a view has validity and is sometimes chosen as the basis of problem-based courses, it is well to remember that problem-based courses also include the context in its broadest sense (social and behavioural, cultural, and planning and administration of health services to meet these needs) to ensure that the needs and problems are set within a relevant framework.

Another criticism is that students' education will be limited to their own personal development and to 'doing a job'. The fear of some is that the broader aspects of education and the scientific basis of what they are doing will be omitted. One would have to agree that this is a reasonable criticism and could be true of some programmes where nursing is conceptualized and practised as a set of tasks, regardless of whether the tasks are cognitive as well as psychomotor. There is a wealth of work being produced at present to show that nursing itself is evolving towards a discipline of study from the earlier models of Donaldson and Crowley (1978), Stevens (1979) and the later work of Benner (1989), Parse (1987), Fawcett (1989), Reed and Procter (1993), Gray and Pratt (1991) and Lumby (1995).

There are several techniques for finding out what students will be required to do as graduates in the workforce. Some of these techniques are major projects and involve time, money and research expertise and are appropriately carried out as part of the planning of an entire curriculum. For example:

- observational techniques for studying current practice by direct observation, video or audiotape; task analysis; situation analysis;
- forecasting techniques for predicting possible future practice priorities; Delphi survey;
- surveying discrete work situations; job description.

To summarize what has been said about the criterion of relevance, the questions to ask and the techniques for answering them are:

Criterion	Questions	Techniques
Relevance	What does the nurse do?	Task analysis
What is the context?	Job description	
What could be expected in the future?	Situation analysis	Future forecasting

LEARNING AND THE LEARNER

The criterion for selecting content based on the student as a learner has not always been recognized in nursing courses. Rather, the selection has been made more often on the basis of its usefulness for immediate practice without consideration of the underlying understanding and principles which would enable its transfer to other situations. Neither is the learner considered when content is chosen and taught on the belief that the information will be needed at some time in the future (Bevis and Watson, 1989).

Considering the student as learner in experience-driven curricula involves responsibilities to teach differently. 'Coming to terms with what is possible to teach the undergraduate is to uncover the complexity and richness of the practice that we want to teach' (Benner, 1989, p 25). Lumby (1995) implies the kind of pathway learners and teachers will tread in 'making visible the knowing involved in the doing . . . perhaps one of our greatest challenges as we return to our practice: to understand what it really means when we talk about "nursing another" and present it for critique'.

Such a speculation raises questions about students and teachers together as learners. Instead of expert givers of information teachers become expert learners. So important are the interactions and transactions between students and students and between students and teachers both focused on learning that Bevis (1989) is prepared to define the curriculum in those terms. In a later chapter we discuss some of the teaching strategies for teaching and learning from experience.

Content for learning implies different goals for the learner than content for action. For example, if you want students to learn by means of their clinical experience placements your expectations of what is to be learned need to be stated as distinct from what you expect the students to do. For example, directing a nurse to give a rationale for the decisions made during crisis care and to trace the sequence of components in decision-making for individual patients, so that future decisions would be based on a recognizable rationale, has vastly different learning implications from simply instructing the nurse to list the decisions made during emergencies.

Applying the criterion of the learner to the selection of content throws the spotlight on the learner's responsibility for meeting her/his own learning needs. This requires skill on the part of the learner; a process to be developed so that dependence on the teacher is reduced. The content of a course is therefore not composed of subject matter only, but process and environment as well.

Another important consideration is the match between the method of learning advocated in the course and the method chosen for nursing practice. Learning and practice are so intertwined that it is important that in choosing content the method of learning does not conflict with the method advocated for practice. For example, if problem-solving is decided to be the relevant learning mode for a particular course, then problem-based practice, or at least the nursing process, would be an appropriate choice for practice so that students would find that learning and practice complemented each other. Choosing to teach about reflective practice requires that time is provided in clinical work to practise the skill of reflection (Woolfolk, 1989).

Again if a certain group of competencies has been identified as the goal for the learner then the choice of content should be guided by the necessary knowledge, skill and attitudes to reach competency. An integrated set of content is required in order that the application to practice is effected and the student is assisted in making further transfer to other situations. Stevens (1979) points to the inconsistencies which plague nursing whereby, for example, a discrete subject- or disease-centred curriculum is taught to students who will use a problem-solving method in practice.

To summarize the criterion of 'Learning and the learner', the following questions and techniques are included:

Criterion	Questions	Techniques
Learning and the learner	What must the nurse know? How will the knowledge be used?	Objectives Competencies Problem-solving

PERSPECTIVE ON NURSING

By now you will probably agree that choosing content for the transmission of nursing knowledge and its translation into practice is a complex task. Most teachers have strong views on what nursing is and what it is not. It is not surprising, then, that teachers often select content on the basis of their perspective on nursing. But, as we have already seen, using one's perspective as the only basis for choice does not always ensure that the resulting content has validity for the full range of activities nurses will perform in many different contexts.

One's perspective may be narrowly confined to the specialties and may not encompass the richness and variety of nursing practice. Moreover, if too specialized, students may not see much relationship between concepts in your specialty and those in other areas of nursing.

Is it possible to express the perspective we hold so that it becomes available to others? A public and not a private perspective? A conceptualization that can be explained through its major and minor concepts? Such a concept map is advocated by Novak and Gowin (1984) and by Heath (1982) for a course which an individual teacher might plan for curricula in nursing, and by Smith (1992) to link theory and basic nursing skills.

Having a perspective on your teaching subject (which, of course, arises out of your beliefs and values) is an important criterion for choosing content. Without it your teaching material will be chosen capriciously and your students will, understandably, be confused about the meaning of nursing as a subject and a service.

What is meant here is a conceptualization of nursing that represents or captures beliefs and values about the meaning of nursing and how it should be practised. How nursing is conceptualized has been the subject of a rapidly mounting literature in recent years. There are many reasons for this. For some writers the main purpose is to identify nursing as a distinctive field of knowledge. For others it is to identify the unique function of the nurse. By clarifying what it is that nurses do (that, if it were not done, no amount of coalescing of the service of other health professionals would replace) the unique function of nurses might be defined. The work of Virginia Henderson is so well known that you will recall immediately the familiar words of her statement on the nature of nursing (1966):

> The unique function of the nurse is to assist the individual, sick or well, in the performance of those activities contributing to health or recovery (or to a peaceful death) that he would perform unaided if he had the necessary strength, will or knowledge. And to do this in such a way as to help him gain independence as rapidly as possible.

Henderson (1991) writes that after 25 years the statement still reflects her concept of the nature of nursing.

All three criteria may now be included in the summary in Table 2.1.

Table 2.1 Criteria and techniques for defining content

Criterion	Questions	Techniques
Relevance	What does the nurse do?	Task analysis
		Job description
	What is the context?	Situation analysis
	What will the nurse do in future?	Future forecasting
Learning and the learner	What must the nurse know?	Objectives
		Competencies
	How will the knowledge be used?	Problem-solving
Perspective of nursing	What view of nursing is held?	Concept mapping
	What kind of person should the nurse be?	Conceptual framework

TECHNIQUES FOR DETERMINING CONTENT

Now that we have explained the background to making decisions about content, we will trace each method to show the steps involved. While the above summary in table form might aid clarification, it also introduces the dangers of over-simplification and arbitrary division of the techniques into categories. There is really a continuum of methods rather than a separation of one technique from another. For example, the links between task analysis, job description, objectives and competencies are fairly direct. Neither are tasks carried out in a vacuum; the context or situation also requires analysis so that the tasks or activities are analysed against their particular set of circumstances.

Taking the criterion of relevance first we will use the techniques listed to answer the questions: what does the nurse do now, in what context, and what will be the future tasks or activities?

ACTIVITY

Imagine that you have been asked to plan a new course in occupational health for primary health-care nurses. You have decided the course should be based on the work students will do when they have completed the course. How will you proceed to define the work?

FEEDBACK

Depending on your experience and knowledge you could begin by finding out:

- What situations?
- What functions?
- What activities?
- What problems?

and finally,

- What knowledge is needed to deal with the problems?

You may be able to supply the answers to all of these questions if you are an experienced occupational health nurse and are therefore familiar with the work conditions and environment in specific situations in occupational health. On the other hand, perhaps you are not up to date with this information, or you may be a community health nurse who has not actually practised in occupational health but has been shouldered with this new responsibility (because of the shortfall of trained occupational health nursing educators). Before planning your course you will need to employ one or more of the following techniques to identify tasks and functions.

TASK ANALYSIS

You may in the first instance choose to consult occupational health nurses for assistance. There are several ways of gaining information in a systematic way:

- by interviewing nurses individually to find out the characteristics of their work – in their own words;
- by asking them to compare an already prepared checklist of task statements with what they actually do;
- by asking them to complete a daily diary sheet by recording what they did throughout each day for several days;
- by inviting a group of occupational health nurses to discuss with you, in an informal meeting, their work and the purposes of their activities; in this way you will gain additional comments about the relative importance to them of the tasks they perform.

Another source of information is the observations you make yourself. There are several ways of observing tasks – from a strictly formalized method to an open 'ethnographic' technique, where the environment and tone of the situation are observed as well as the tasks. You could:

- conduct a time and motion study to obtain a quantitative record of how occupational nurses spend their time;
- choose a number of broad categories beforehand (e.g. interpersonal interaction, treatment, advising) then observe the particular activities carried out in each category;
- become involved in occupational health work yourself, as a participant observer, collecting your impressions as well as the more objective evidence of what tasks and activities are performed in the job;
- collect a number of incidents of both excellent and unsatisfactory performances which could be used as critical incidents in compiling details of what the nurse must do and know.

Another technique involves your students and becomes part of their initial project in a problem-solving or in a self-directed study course.

You could:

- design a project with your students to enable them to find out for themselves the elements of the work they will need to understand in order to perform later on.

The outcome of any of the above methods will be a set of information which you can then organize into levels of activities, tasks or functions. Starting with the information gained from any of these methods of task analysis, it is a simple step to form a job description.

Job description: Category – Occupational Health Nurse

General situation in which the occupational health nurse will work

The occupational health nurse is responsible for the health of workers in the plant. There is a medical officer in the district to whom referrals can be made.

Functions

1. Conduct safety promotion programmes
2. Evaluate hazards specific to industry
3. Supervise environmental monitoring
4. Assist workers to help themselves to deal with day-to-day crises.

Sample of activities within the functions

1. Conduct safety promotion programmes:
   (a) interview workers to assess possible allergies
   (b) advise on occupational hazards specific to industry
   (c) select personal protective devices
   (d) fit personal safety equipment.
2. Evaluate hazards specific to industry:
   (a) apply knowledge of these hazards to work environment
   (b) monitor occupational hazards
   (c) notify hazardous levels of the work environment to authorities.
   . . . and so on.

Each of the activities can be subdivided into more specific tasks if the level of detail you require (and your purposes in teaching the course) demands more precision in the definition of tasks. There is a great variety in the amount of detail contained in job descriptions. The rule of thumb here is simply to decide on the amount of specificity you require to assist you in deciding what to teach. (This will depend on many associated factors such as length of the course, what the students know already, what resources you have and the extent to which your colleagues in the occupational health field can assist you with on-site demonstration and field experiences.)

By now it should be fairly obvious that task analysis (narrowly employed) should not be undertaken in isolation from the constraints or the resources in the practice setting where teaching is to take place. After all, the quantitative method of task analysis reveals what is done but not what is omitted.

LEARNING OBJECTIVES

The importance of an analysis of tasks is that from it a set of learning objectives can be developed. The questions – 'What does the nurse do?' and 'What must the nurse learn?' – lead to the formation of a learning objective, i.e. those things students must know or be able to do at the completion of the course.

ACTIVITY

In view of the controversy about the usefulness of learning objectives and competencies, would you consider omitting altogether the step of constructing learning objectives now that you have a job description of the work occupational health nurses do to assist you to choose content for your course? What implications arise from the additional step of forming a set of learning objectives? Make a list of pros and cons.

FEEDBACK

This would make a fruitful topic for debate as the issues range throughout general education (Raths, 1971; Stenhouse, 1975; Brady, 1992), medical education (Simpson, 1980; Engel, 1980) and nursing education (Stevens, 1979; Gibson, 1980; Martin and Sheehan, 1985; Sheehan and Sheehan, 1985; Crotty, 1989; Quinn, 1994).

Your pros and cons list might contain some of the following points:

Pro objectives
- Directs the learner.
- Directs the teacher.
- States the behaviour to be achieved.

- Assists in selecting content.
- Enables sequencing of content.
- Aids measurement of achievement.

Con objectives
- Too limiting.
- Trivializes behaviour.
- Describes observable behaviour only.
- Outcomes of learning difficult to predict.
- Neglects interaction of cognitive, psychomotor and affective objectives. Could overlook spontaneity in classroom.

For our purposes in this chapter, it would be difficult (as Stenhouse (1975) admits) to deny the usefulness of objectives because they communicate to students, other teachers and practitioners what it is that students need to learn. This may seem a contradiction at first sight; we are trying to determine what to teach yet we are stating content in terms of what students must learn.

If we take a simple example the difference between a learning objective and a teaching objective can be illustrated.

- **Learning objective**: On completion of instruction the student will be able to identify the hazards caused by different toxicity levels in a given environment.
- **Teacher objective**: To ensure that students understand the hazards of different toxicity levels.

The first statement shows what the student must do and under what circumstances. Assessment to see whether the student is competent can be carried out. On the other hand the second objective relates to what the teacher will do and it is not at all clear what expectations of student performance will be required. Understandably, students and possibly the teacher will be unsure or even confused.

In summary, in order to write learning objectives, simply take each of the tasks from the job description and restate them in the form of what the student must know, be able to do, or what attitudes the student should exhibit, in order to perform the task satisfactorily and show that she/he is competent.

Before leaving the topic of objectives, it is important to consider the arguments about learning objectives in nursing at present. Heath and Marson (1979) point out the pitfalls inherent in trying to describe the more elusive but worthwhile behaviour we require of students. Stevens (1979) points to the pressures to 'cover' content, which tends to relegate content to two of the lowest levels of cognitive skills, recall and recognition. Reilly (1980) presents objectives from the perspective of the nursing process so that the stages of Assessment, Planning, Intervention and Evaluation have learning objectives that generalize across many different patient-care problems, while Quinn (1994) gives examples of objectives at all taxonomic levels of the cognitive, affective and psychomotor scales.

One final but important comment is appropriate: that is that the decision to use or not use objectives relates to the curriculum design and structure of the total course. If, for example, the course is to feature mastery learning then objectives are required to enable criterion-referenced assessment of mastery to be accomplished. Stating clinical learning objectives enables a distinction to be made between what is required to be done (e.g. to conduct an interview) and what is required to be learnt as a result of the doing (e.g. to compare your progress in interviewing using a prepared learning guide).

It may be helpful to pause at this point to review the progress we have made in answering the questions related to relevance in Table 2. 1.

Only one question, 'What does the nurse do?', has been addressed. But by exploring the techniques of task analysis and job description that could be used to answer that question, we found that the criterion of the learner and learning was also involved – 'What must the nurse know?'

SITUATION ANALYSIS

Returning to the criterion of relevance and the question 'What is the context?', we are reminded that professional performance does not occur within a vacuum. There is no mystery here, if the client, the task and the setting are considered together. Moreover, the tasks and functions identified through observation (or any of the other methods) need to be regarded as part of the environment in which they are performed. Take the illustration of the occupational health nurse once more. It would be ludicrous to accept a list of tasks to be performed without a description of the environment, because they interact with each other.

For example, 'identifying the hazards caused by toxic agents' involves not only a measurement of toxicity levels and a knowledge of their harmful effects but also the awareness of anxiety levels of workers, the heating, lighting and ventilation of the plant and also whether the pattern of communication of workers and management is co-operative or confrontational.

COMPETENCY

At once the question will arise, 'How does this assist me to decide what I am to teach?' Laduca (1975) has constructed a grid called 'professional competence situation universe' where a three-dimensional model is used to depict the client, the clinical problem and the setting. Gonczi,

Haager and Oliver (1990) contribute another model with three key elements: attributes, performance and standards. Knowledge, abilities, skills and attitudes make up the attributes of competence and we can say that a competency combines the attributes that underlie professional performance which is assessed according to clearly set standards.

Both the approaches described above make possible the integration of three components instead of treating each one as a separate subject. Using Laduca's model a number of situations are chosen and the relevant content about the client, the problem and the setting is identified. For example, taking the objective 'identify the hazards caused by different toxicity levels' a situation where factory workers are exposed to toxic fumes during the manufacture of rubber tyres would be identified. The situation would be described in full, the characteristics of the workers and the setting included and the problem of the hazards of toxic gas would be determined.

The difficulty arises when competencies are so broad that it becomes difficult to determine what the student is to know, to do and to be. This is a particular concern for clinical teachers, who may be left to determine what skills the competency requires and could, therefore, be in doubt as to what to teach. There are important consequences , as Pratt (1989, p 20) has observed, since the profession expects that its graduates will be able to perform 'the requisite behavioural repertoire'.

ACTIVITY

Taking the occupational health example once more, develop a competency from the information below:

Activity	Client	Situation	Problems
Identify hazards caused by different toxicity levels	All employees	Small factory	Absenteeism
		Sympathetic management	Fatigue
			Depression

FEEDBACK

A competency, or the ability to perform a set of activities, or to enact a role adequately or effectively is based on an integration of content. The characteristics of the client, the description of the immediate surroundings and events, the goal to be achieved and the standard of performance to be reached are all part of the competency. That is to say that situations rather than academic subjects are the basis for deciding what to teach.

It is possible to devise a set of competencies to cover the situations a competent nurse must be prepared to manage and then select the content that must be learned and practised.

In the chosen example a suggested competency would be:

- **Competency**: Collect, analyse and report on data pertaining to toxicity levels, employee exposure and health, and report results with recommendations to the appropriate authority.

FUTURE FORECASTING

Many nurse teachers believe that it is not enough to develop content on the basis of current practice, that relevance extends to preparing the graduates of a course to have a knowledge of present and future health care and health-care trends. Deciding what to teach in this case needs a different technique from those we have already discussed.

ACTIVITY

Imagine you have been invited to provide a projection of what will be required by occupational health nurses in the future. The company has decided to expand its operation and to diversify its activities. The manager has said he requires nurses who will meet the challenges of the future and wants you to set up a continuing education course. How will you decide what to teach?

FEEDBACK

Perhaps the first thing you would do is to interview the company's management and planning departments to ascertain the time constraints they are working in. You could also seek information on the type of diversification of activities they are planning and the goals they have set.

Armed with that information you could then select a number of experts to form a sample for a future forecasting exercise. The sample could contain occupational health nurses, community nurses, company personnel, health department and nurse education representatives.

Bevis (1982) viewed current health-care trends in the light of predictions about changes in society and society's way of coping, and drew up a detailed forecast of possible changes in the future. This was then used as a basis for selection of content.

A technique known as Delphi Probe (Sullivan and Brye, 1983) can be used. The Delphi technique is a tool using sequential questionnaires. After the first round of questionnaires have been returned, the responses are analysed, coalesced and returned to the same sample for the next round of questions. Repeating this once more, the final responses reveal the crystallized opinions of the experts. Beddome *et al.* (1995) used a Delphi technique to ascertain from practitioners what they believed the nurse of the future needed to do, to know and to be.

An important point is made by Bevis (1982), who points out that it is still necessary to clarify what activities or behaviours the forecasted future changes will require in order to select specific content and experiences.

The Delphi survey technique used to select content can be summarized as a number of steps:

- ask experts about projected changes;
- recycle answers to the same experts;
- repeat twice (or at least once);
- compile the end results into future forecasts;
- identify tasks, activities, functions, behaviours;
- select content.

PROBLEM-SOLVING

How will the student use the knowledge that she/he must know? Referring back to Table 2.1 we nominated problem-solving as an appropriate technique. (Actually, in attempting a full answer to the question, we are in deep water and the issues raised by such a question are treated in Chapter 3.) So, in this chapter, we are looking at problem-solving as a way of determining what to teach.

ACTIVITY

You are planning to use the problem-solving method in teaching your students. What advantages do you see in using this method in deciding content for your course?

FEEDBACK

If you are teaching in a problem-based course, naturally your students will use a problem-based method of learning. For a detailed discussion see Barrows and Tamblyn, 1980; Boud and Feletti, 1991; Higgins, 1994. The Barrows and Tamblyn text is written by a physician and a nurse; the text deals with the development and implementation of the method.

Disadvantages, you might have noted, are inherent in a problem-solving method that has become 'de-problemized'. Geach (1974) pointed out what she believed to be an intellectualizing of problem-solving. Students were taught a method that had little reflection in day-to-day dealing with real problems. Her view in 'The problem-solving technique: is it relevant to nursing practice?' was aimed at bringing teachers and clinicians together to resolve the dilemma.

Another disadvantage you might have come across is the weakening of the students' opportunity to learn through problem-solving by prescribing beforehand what pathway should be followed. This is a considerable curtailment of initiative (and is antithetical to problem-solving) if it is applied in the form of a checklist to every patient.

Yet another disadvantage to learning to nurse occurs when the problem-solving method is used to rehearse the student's responses before there is an opportunity for applying problem-solving in the real situation.

Allen (1977) shows two ways of teaching in the problem-solving mode.

- Students can be prepared beforehand to meet several situations.
- The teacher can provide the means by which the student and patient can interact together in a problem-solving way.

An example of the first method is where teacher and student rehearse what will be said to the patient, possible replies by the patient and how the patient will be prepared. Allen comments that 'training a nurse to respond to artificial situations of this nature is in conflict with the problem-solving approach' (p 28). The alternative suggested by Allen is the second method, where nurses learn to nurse patients whose problems are less well known and understood (see Allen for a detailed account of the two types of teaching).

Returning to the original intent of this section – determining content using the problem-solving method – and using problem-solving as in the second method above, it is apparent that the student and the patient, not the teacher, determine the content. The content is not prescribed beforehand but is identified by the student, who realizes what information they require after interviewing, or discussing how the patient views the problem. In determining content, the student learns to distinguish important from less important material and also where or from whom the information may be obtained. In effect the student learns what knowledge and skills are required and how they will use that knowledge and skill.

ACTIVITY

Not all problem-solving can be taught on-site with the patient or client. In classroom teaching, what content would you be able to supply?

FEEDBACK

Again, the student will determine most of the content in a true problem-solving method. The teacher provides the resources.

For example, a computer-assisted programme could be used where the student gives alternative responses to meet the problem.

Another set of resources can be supplied in the form of a patient study, where a patient's initial history and record is supplied. The student then determines what additional information is required.

A third method is an 'in-basket' set of materials, where the material relevant to a problem is supplied. The student must identify the problem(s), give a rationale and a set of actions to be used in the resolution. Examples of resource materials are community situations such as:

- the local council's ruling in respect of housing;
- a disadvantaged resident's letter to the daily paper;
- a domiciliary nurse's report on a terminally ill patient in the housing affected;
- a letter to the local hospital from the patient's family asking for increased resources;

and so on.

For the teacher, the selection of content becomes the selection of resources.

CONCEPT MAPPING

What view of nursing is held? What kind of person should the nurse be? These questions are related to the criterion we named 'having a perspective on nursing' in order to determine content for teaching.

A concept map is a way of representing the central ideas within a field of knowledge or a discipline of study. By drawing a map that links the concepts (or main ideas, or points of interest) the relationship among the concepts can be linked and described. It is the linking of the concepts which is of great interest to nurses at present. As we shall see later in this section, stating the relationship between two concepts is a way of forming a principle.

In nurse education a framework made up of concepts and principles (or a conceptual framework) serves two important purposes: first, as a basis for curriculum development and for the selection of content, teaching methods and modes of practice; second, as a basis for the development of nursing theory. When the principles (or propositions) are tested the conceptual framework then becomes a theoretical framework and from it begins the development of a theory.

For our purposes, in this text we are interested in concept mapping as a stimulus for generating content for a course, and on a smaller scale for a lesson. Additionally, by using the method of concept mapping students are able themselves to identify the relationships between concepts and to begin to generate principles which they will later test for their application to practice. Concept mapping is, therefore, not only a way of determining content but a method of learning to transfer knowledge into practice.

Why not try constructing a concept map step by step in order to trace the features and process of developing a map?

ACTIVITY

Imagine you are planning a new set of teaching/learning sessions on rehabilitation and you want your students to realize the continuous nature of rehabilitation, its multidisciplinary character and the extension of its principle throughout the patients' progress to the home, family and work. What main ideas would you select as the core concepts for the course?

FEEDBACK

Your list of ideas may have included the following:

- Self-concept
- Prevention
- Mobility

- Independence
- Interpersonal growth
- Adaptation
- Family/friends
- Values
- Quality of life.

It is often helpful to ask a few colleagues to do the same, or together 'brainstorm' ideas about rehabilitation and add any new concepts to the list such as:

- Structural changes
- Body image
- Facing reality
- Learning
- Change
- Building on positives
- Honesty
- Wheelchair
- Prosthesis
- Decision-making
- Self-help
- Cost-effectiveness
- Security (economic)
- Coping with limitations
- Rehabilitation aids.

When you have exhausted the ideas, identify the most and least inclusive concepts. Proceeding with concept mapping, link the concepts in hierarchy from most inclusive to least inclusive and state any relationships you recognize.

One way of linking the concepts is illustrated in Figure 2.1.

If you are satisfied that the concept map represents your major concept and the required flow of ideas, you could then identify the content and practice you wish to teach.

Rehabilitation is an interesting area for concept mapping as the role of the nurse is often unclear and because of this the teaching of rehabilitation is often limited to the domain of other health professionals. Clearly, there is a role for nursing in rehabilitation. But identifying content by conventional means, e.g. psychology, sociology, orthopaedics or gerontology, fails to highlight concepts of learning, decision-making, quality of life – all arising from the needs of the person and the situation rather than the professional or the academic discipline.

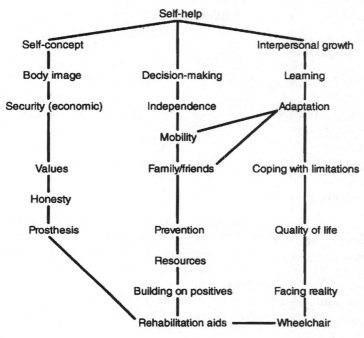

Figure 2.1   Example of a concept hierarchy map.

SUMMARY

Deciding what to teach, as we have seen in this chapter, can be a complex task for a teacher.

Any one of a number of methods can be used to determine the content of your teaching. Content in the broadest sense, including knowledge, skills and attitudes, is what is meant and sometimes a combination of several methods will assist you to achieve the aims of your course. Your particular purpose in assisting students to learn to nurse, and your personal style as a teacher and as a practitioner of nursing, will also determine your choice of method of determining what you will teach.

As a summary of the main points we have discussed in this chapter, why not try the final activity.

ACTIVITY

Make a list of the purposes for which you would use each of the following techniques for determining content:

- Task analysis
- Job description
- Situation analysis
- Future forecasting
- Objectives
- Competencies
- Problem-solving
- Concept mapping.

FEEDBACK

It is possible that your list will be different from the list any of your colleagues might produce in answer to the same activity. There are no right or wrong answers. However, inappropriate use of some techniques could result in a selection of content for your course that fails to satisfy you or your students. Again your knowledge of the level and progress of your students and your appreciation of the aims of the total course will influence your choice of method. The following, therefore, is meant only as a guide.

Use task analysis if you aim to:

- base your teaching on specific components of nursing practice, e.g. demonstrations;
- develop specific behavioural objectives for your students;
- identify the knowledge, skills and attitudes in a particular activity;
- identify components of the nurse's role in total patient care.

Use situational analysis if you aim to:

- include the context and the environment of nursing activities in your course;
- emphasize to students the importance of the patient's background (e.g. family and work) in the planning for and giving of care;
- base your selection of content on the problems of patients rather than a series of separated subjects.

Use job description if you aim to:

- determine the specific steps in a task or activity;
- provide the student with the elements of the work they will be required to do;
- direct your teaching towards the tasks and activities expected of your students.

Use future forecasting if you aim to:

- plan a course to meet the future as well as the immediate needs of students;
- prepare students for change;
- stimulate your teaching by keeping up to date with trends in your field.

Use objectives if you aim to:

- specify a number of levels of achievement expected of students;
- provide a learning guide to students;
- define the limits of the course;
- provide criteria for assessment.

Use competencies if you aim to:

- include qualitative as well as quantitative dimensions of care;
- provide a basis for interdisciplinary content;
- include sets of activities to be achieved rather than specific tasks;
- provide for integration of tasks and clinical situations.

Use problem-solving if you aim to:

- complement the general aims of a problem-based course;
- prepare students for problem-based nursing practice;
- involve students in determining what they need to know in resolving problems.

Use concept mapping if you aim to:

- identify a set of concepts to represent a patient problem;
- cut across subject boundaries;
- integrate knowledge from several fields;
- present nursing knowledge so that it transfers to practice.

Helping students learn 3

INTRODUCTION

The purpose of this chapter is to examine some aspects of learning theory which are relevant to the education of nurses.

When you have finished this chapter you should be able to use relevant aspects of learning theories as the basis for decisions about the way you arrange your teaching to help students learn.

There are many excellent books that deal with specific theories of learning or which integrate or provide overviews of the major theories. It is not possible within a single chapter to deal with the details and the interrelationships of those theories. The purpose of this chapter is, therefore, to sketch an outline of current beliefs about how students learn and to provide a framework for decisions teachers make. References will be provided throughout and are recommended if you wish to follow up any aspects more thoroughly.

Aspects of specific teaching methods which are frequently used in nurse education are discussed in the following chapter, and it is true that most teachers operate within a context of traditional teaching methods such as lectures, practical classes of some sort and small-group work. However, even within those traditional methods there is room for innovation and application of ideas intended to maximize the learning students experience. The first step toward such innovations is for teachers to ask themselves 'How do students learn?' and to base their teaching on the answers to that question. You do not have to be an expert in educational theory to answer that question. All teachers have also been students for considerable periods of time and have experienced both effective and ineffective learning episodes. So the answer to the question 'How do students learn?' begins with your own experiences.

ACTIVITY

Think about your learning career as a nursing student and as a graduate. Can you remember a learning experience which was particularly effective? What made it effective? Write down as many things about it as you can remember.

Sometimes it is easier to recall learning experiences that did not work well – is there some topic that you always found difficult? How were you taught about that topic; what factors inhibited your learning? Write down what you feel are the reasons you were unable to learn effectively.

FEEDBACK

Obviously there can be no 'model feedback' for this activity because learning is a personal experience and not all learners will require the same conditions for learning. In fact that is one of the most important things for teachers to remember – there are differences among students which affect their learning.

The factors you have listed might include factors within yourself which influenced your ability or readiness to learn, factors within the environment or context or factors within the subject matter itself which helped or hindered your learning. It is artificial to separate conditions for learning into discrete categories since there is considerable interaction between personal, contextual and topic characteristics; however, for ease of presentation these categories will be used as the basic organizing structure for the remainder of this chapter. It will become clear as we proceed that there is considerable overlap among the factors discussed, and some concepts, such as motivation and feedback for example, feature in all categories.

CONDITIONS FOR LEARNING – WITHIN THE STUDENT

ACTIVITY

Drawing on your experience as a learner and a teacher, identify the major factors within the individual that influence learning.

FEEDBACK

Factors within the student which may influence learning are numerous. Your list might include the following:

- motivation to learn;
- interest in the topic;
- general ability or intelligence;
- aptitude for the topic or specific skills;
- learning style or preferred learning strategies.

You may also have listed other factors, or used different terms from the ones used here. There is some overlap between the abstract concepts that have been developed to define individual differences among learners. For example, the unitary concept of intelligence as measured by intelligence testing reflects motivation, general abilities, specific skills, cognitive strategies and cultural differences. Similarly 'personality tests' measure aspects of abilities, motivation, strategies, preferences and cultural characteristics. The important thing to remember about such definitions of individual differences is that, while they are concepts that may be useful in planning learning experiences which accommodate to individual needs, they are usually not sufficiently precise or reliable to be used as predictors of student performance. Allocation of tertiary level students to 'ability groups' may be convenient for the teacher but the benefits for the students are debatable. While prescription of specific remedial activities may enhance certain aspects of the students' performance, other aspects of ability grouping reinforce teachers' lowered expectations of lower-level groups and poor self-concepts of students in those groups, resulting in a 'self-fulfilling prophecy' which may actually impede the progress of those students.

Individual differences contribute to students' opportunities to learn from each other and they present a challenge to teachers who are interested in getting to know their students and in helping each student to maximize her/his learning potential.

Good teaching triggers the intellectual and motivational resources of each student. A particular topic or style of teaching may be exciting to some and boring to others, but the meaning gained from pages read, lectures heard, observations made in the laboratory or in the field, and actions taken in the clinic or studio derives from each student's distinctive meld of cognitive and affective capabilities.

(Ericksen, 1985, quoting from Hunt, 1983)

The nature of individual differences is extremely complex and attempts to develop general rules to assist teachers in linking specific teaching strategies with specific individual abilities have met with limited success despite considerable research efforts. Nevertheless, teachers will be assisted by a general awareness of the nature of individual differences and their potential influence on learning.

MOTIVATION

Motivation can be defined in many ways but for our purposes we will take it to mean the desire or wish to learn. The desire to learn can be generated by many factors, some of which are more relevant for some students and some learning contexts than others.

ACTIVITY

What motivates your students to learn what you teach them?
    What motivates you to continue your professional learning?
    Do your reasons for wanting to learn differ from those of your students in any significant ways? What makes the difference, if there is one?

FEEDBACK

The list of factors that motivate individuals to learn is endless and very dependent on specific circumstances; however, one important distinction can be made which provides a framework for understanding the nature of motivation, that is the distinction between a desire to learn generated from within the individual and a desire to learn generated by external influences.

Traditional educational programmes provide quite a high degree of external motivation in the form of barrier examinations, grades, rules for admission to and exclusion from courses, and expressions of praise or criticism from teachers. By contrast, internal motivation arises in situations where the learner has an intrinsic interest in the learning task, pursuing personal educational goals to increase a sense of personal mastery and professional competence. While the two types of motivation are certainly not mutually exclusive, teachers frequently observe that students 'are only interested in what they will be asked in the exams'. New students begin with a degree of internal motivation to learn to be competent nurses, but the facts of survival teach them that such goals are a subordinate issue to passing examinations and pleasing the teachers, and external motivation gradually takes precedence for most students. Once the students have graduated and become practising professionals, however, most of the external imperative to learn is removed and graduates must rediscover their sources of internal motivation in order to maintain professional competence. Some do so quite successfully but some have been so disenchanted with learning to pass the examinations that they have little desire to continue their learning and seek only enough professional education to keep them safe.

In the above activity you may have noticed that your reasons for learning are related to your personal needs and responsibilities, while to some extent at least your students' reasons for learning are related to the requirement to satisfy external conditions before personal needs or interests. The task for teachers is to create conditions for learning in which students' internal motivation is recognized and encouraged to develop, and in which sources of external motivation are kept in proper perspective.

While it may be true that 'students learn what they care about and remember what they understand' (Ericksen, 1985, p 51), the research-based concepts of reinforcement and curiosity can motivate and stimulate students' interest in learning.

There are strong links in the work of early psychologists Pavlov, Hull, Thorndike and, later, Skinner, in developing the concept of reinforcement and in showing the power of reward and punishment as motivators. Although the behaviourist and reductionist emphasis in the concept when applied to testing and assessment in nursing is now controversial, the basic principles are still useful. For example, the principle of schedules of reinforcement has been shown to assist the learning of skills when reinforcement is given once in a while, not every time the performance is correct (the patient fisherman phenomenon). 'Material learned under conditions of aperiodic reinforcement remains in memory better than if it were learned under constant or regular reinforcement' (Ericksen, 1985, p 45). The power of rewards (for example, in terms of praise) over punishment (in terms of 'put-downs') in motivating the learner is well known and confirmed in the research studies on reinforcement. For teachers it is even more important to realize that 'either praise or blame is more effective in promoting learning than ignoring a student's efforts' (Fraenkel, 1980). The 'carrot and stick' method is really extrinsic to the student, while self-reinforcement in reading, or in setting oneself a challenging task so that gaining understanding becomes its own reward, is intrinsic.

Maslow (1943) proposed a theory of motivation which is a useful conceptual framework. He suggested a hierarchy of five basic needs beginning with the need for physiological satisfaction and progressing through the needs for safety, love, self-esteem and self-actualization. Comparison of sources of motivation in nursing education with this hierarchy reveals that the external motivation described above relates mainly to the need for safety and to some extent the need for 'love' or approval from one's teachers and colleagues. Internal motivation as described above relates more closely to the need for self-esteem, which leads to a feeling of self-confidence, worth and capability, and to the need for self-actualization – the process by which one comes to depend on the self rather than to identify with others and to rely, when necessary, on personal standards independently of external demands (Lovell, 1980, p 111). Given this definition, self-actualization is clearly to be encouraged in the education of nurses.

INTEREST IN THE TOPIC

Interest in the topic to be learned is related to motivation and the desire to learn. It is inevitable that levels of interest will vary among students, who will be influenced by a multitude of factors such as personal preferences and abilities, like or dislike of the teacher, the presence of competing events such as examinations in another subject, or even the time of day or season. You may have little control over some of these factors that impinge on the students' interest; however, a major factor that you can do something about is the perceived relevance of what the students have to learn. Pressured by competing demands on their time, students have to make decisions about learning priorities – one criterion they use to help them decide is relevance. Students judge the relevance of a topic according to how well they can perceive a relationship between that topic and their ultimate goal of becoming a nurse. Consequently, ward work is seen to be very relevant and generates a lot of interest. Basic science courses, when taught in isolation from clinical practice or examples, have a more tenuous relationship to the ultimate goal and are perceived as less relevant hurdles to be surmounted rather than integral parts of nursing education. Teachers can increase the perceived relevance of topics at any stage of training by attention to the sequence in which subject matter is presented. For example, traditional structures of disciplines tend to progress from basic facts to combinations of those facts into general principles and then application of those principles in solution of problems. Not surprisingly, teachers often follow this same sequence in their teaching because it is logical and familiar; unfortunately it may be less motivating and interesting for the students, who cannot grasp the relevance of the basic facts and principles until they have experienced the problems to which those facts and principles will be applied. Problem-based learning experiences and inquiry-based learning (Feletti, 1993), methods of linking theory and practice (Smith, 1992), vertical integration of subjects and conceptual frameworks based on a nursing model, are all attempts to use alternative approaches to the sequence of instruction which demonstrate relevance and promote interest. At a more basic level, asking students questions or giving them problems to solve stimulates curiosity and generates more interest than does merely providing information as a collection of facts.

GENERAL ABILITY OR INTELLIGENCE

While general ability or intelligence in its general sense undoubtedly influences the capacity of individuals to learn, the specific effects are impossible to determine simply because we have no adequate definitions or criteria for such general abilities (Lovell, 1980, p 99). Individuals differ in their innate potential for learning along innumerable dimensions and although there may be marked differences in a group of students, some educators believe that, given appropriate learning experiences, 'all or almost all students can master what they are taught' (Block, 1971, p 3). This should certainly be true in nursing education where a selection process has been used to decide which students will be accepted for training. In professional training courses, where academic performance is invariably one criterion used for selection, teachers have few grounds for attributing poor student performance to 'lack of ability'.

APTITUDES AND SPECIFIC SKILLS

Aptitudes and specific skills are components of general ability that are capable of being identified and defined. To a certain extent they may be innate but they are also certainly shaped by training and experience. For example, innate musical talent may differentiate the concert pianist from the mediocre player, but no amount of innate talent will create a concert pianist from someone who begins musical training late in life. Some nursing schools have attempted to identify specific aptitudes and skills which are believed essential in the profession of nursing and, where possible, to incorporate those into selection procedures. Ability to communicate effectively is one such aptitude. On the other hand, some aptitudes are expected to develop during the education and clinical programme and become part of the learning objectives rather than criteria for selection.

ACTIVITY

Which aptitudes or specific skills do you expect students to exhibit or develop in the area that you teach? What difficulties do students encounter in achieving those objectives? Do some achieve the desirable level of skill faster than others?

FEEDBACK

The last question in that activity is a leading question, since one conception of aptitude defines it as the characteristic which predicts the rate at which a student can learn a given task, rather than the level of learning possible. Out of this idea developed the concept of mastery learning, which proposes that, discounting 5% of individuals with specific disabilities for certain subjects, 95% of students can learn a subject to a high level of mastery if given sufficient learning time and appropriate types of help. Some students will require more effort, time and help to achieve the criterion level or the level of minimum competence required. The teacher's task is to find ways of reducing the learning time for slower students so that it does not become prohibitively slow, and to offer enrichment experiences for those students who proceed at a faster pace (Bloom, 1971).

Mastery learning is a very important concept in nursing education where professional responsibilities demand that all registered nurses have achieved at least a minimum level of competence in central aspects of their role. Core curricula define those competencies which students must master and the level of satisfactory performance. Once those objectives have been achieved students can progress to develop skills and knowledge in 'should know' areas, then 'nice to know' areas (Abbatt, 1992).

Aptitudes for learning in specific areas are not static and may progress with the development of the individual; maintaining and strengthening necessary aptitudes is therefore a factor that teachers should consider in deciding how to help students learn (Cronbach and Snow, 1977). Flexibility needs to be built into learning experiences to allow for differential rates of progress and different levels of need for information or practice. One approach to providing this flexibility is the use of self-paced modules or learning units, which allow students to progress through subject matter at their own speed and to use their contact with the teacher for higher level learning such as comprehension, critical thinking and problem-solving. The Open University units, the modules developed for the *Nursing Times* (1991) and those developed for distance learning are good examples.

A related factor, which teachers should bear in mind, is the 'readiness' of students to undertake learning in certain areas. Readiness may relate to aptitudes, previous experience, interest or personal development and it is to be expected that various levels of readiness will exist among students and that learning experiences may have to take account of that variation. Tight (1983, p 55) shows that adults' readiness to learn is intertwined with the developmental tasks of their social roles and that their 'time perspective changes from one of postponed application of knowledge to immediacy of application, and accordingly (their) orientation toward learning shifts from one of subject-centredness to one of problem-centredness'. For example, some students may be ready to deal with factual issues before emotional issues, some students may need to deal with emotional issues before they can address the technical or factual issues. Not all students may be ready to take part in a discussion about care of the dying patient so the discussion should be structured in a way which allows an atmosphere of comfort and trust and which introduces the topic at a level which is meaningful to all participants. Experienced teachers, like experienced nurses, can call on their professional judgement to help them analyse the situation and formulate a management plan, on the spot if necessary.

There are no hard and fast rules to help teachers adapt teaching to students' individual needs, since too many variables intervene to allow accurate prescription of strategies. However, if you are aware of, and sensitive to, the variations in readiness and aptitudes which occur even within an academically homogeneous group you will maintain sufficient flexibility to help all your students learn and achieve the required level of competence.

LEARNING STYLE AND STRATEGIES

Learning style (sometimes called cognitive style) is a concept of individual differences which is relevant to education. Cognitive style is basically the ways in which people process information. It incorporates such things as the ways in which sensory stimuli are perceived and interpreted, the strategy that the individual uses in forming concepts and solving problems, and the approaches an individual takes to learning a given body of material. For example, some people tend to gather information systematically and arrive at solutions to problems by logical deduction (focusing), while other people tend to begin with a few educated guesses and gather information as they proceed (scanning) (Bruner, Goodnow and Austin, 1956); some seek a single right or best answer to questions or problems (convergers), while some prefer to cast the net widely, seeking potential solutions in innovative areas (divergers). Hudson (1968) has described 'syllabus-bound' learners who happily accept the restrictions of a formal syllabus and aim for good examination results, and 'syllabus-free' learners who have intellectual interests extending beyond the set syllabus. Pask (1976) has categorized learning strategies as serialist – in which the learner prefers to build up a total picture by accumulating and assembling details, and holist – in which the learner prefers to gain an overview of the topic as a general structure in which the details fall into place. Kagan (1965) has observed that some learners, when confronted with a problem, delay before offering a solution which is usually correct – they take the time to internally evaluate potential solutions. Kagan called this 'reflectivity'. In contrast, some learners offer solutions rapidly which are often wrong, relying on the teacher or some other external source to evaluate their efforts: this tendency was designated 'impulsivity'. Marton and Saljo (1984) described a 'deep approach' to learning taken by students where there is an active search for meaning, and a 'surface approach' where the student relies on memorizing. A good review of the individual differences in cognitive styles is available in Biggs and Telfer (1983).

Ramsden (1988) claims that the perspective students have on learning influences how and what will be learned. This kind of learning is different from knowing facts and principles and from carrying out a procedure. The emphasis is on how the learner uses knowledge to interpret a phenomenon – for example, understanding principles from social and behavioural sciences so that they can be applied to a clinical situation, rather than simply learning the details of principles for assessment and examination purposes.

Rather than applying psychological theories to students' learning in a 'top-down' manner, Biggs (1989) indicates that studying 'students in context', inductively bottom-up, is a more productive way of discovering how students learn. As a result, learning is more likely to be studied from the learner's point of view than from that of the researcher or teacher.

A critical study of the details of these dimensions of cognitive styles may lead to the suspicion that many researchers are using different terms to describe very similar tendencies which overlap considerably with older notions such as creativity, intelligence and personality variables. Nevertheless, the dimensions do offer some insights into the complexities involved in perceiving, processing and retaining information in a form in which it is able to be used effectively. Without a doubt, learners are very active in the process of learning.

Learning 'is an active process of mind on experience' (Wilson, 1981, p 25). By contrast, many traditional teaching strategies such as lectures and tests of factual recall are based on a passive model of learning in which 'knowledge as a copy of reality ... has to be committed in its present form to the memory of the learner' (Wilson, 1981, p 24). Piaget (1971) described learning as essentially a simultaneous process of assimilation and accommodation in which the learner incorporates the learned object or event while also taking account of its peculiarities and adapting existing cognitive structures to achieve a good fit. Ausubel (1960) extended this idea with the suggestion that learning can be improved by the provision of 'advance organizers', which help the student to activate relevant parts of his or her cognitive structures in readiness for the assimilation and accommodation which forms the crucial part of the learning task.

The following activity will provide an example of what is meant by advance organizers.

ACTIVITY

Read this list of syllables and then close your eyes and try to recall as many as you can: MAI, CON, DEL, MAR, MAS, PEN, RHO, VER, GEO, FLO, VIR.

FEEDBACK

Probably you tried to make some sense out of the syllables as an aid to memory. Given the task of learning nonsense syllables people usually try to link them to words or link them together into meaningful sentences or work out some type of code to fit into their memory (or cognitive structure). In fact these syllables are the first three letters of the names of 11 states on the east coast of the USA. If you had known that at the beginning would you have found it easier to learn the list? Probably your answer is 'yes'. If you had been given that advance organizer you would have been able to call up the relevant parts of your existing knowledge and fit the new learning into it in a way which would have facilitated your ability to recall the syllables. The advance organizer would have transformed the syllables from meaningless to meaningful information.

What does this mean for the teacher? It means that learning will only occur if the subject or skill or attitude to be learned has meaning for the student and can be fitted into what the student already knows from education or experience. Learning that cannot be locked into existing knowledge or cognitive structure is short-lived and may not be retained in usable form. Once again, however, individual differences among students will create problems for the teacher who cannot be expected to know which learning styles are preferred by which students, nor which aspects of the learning are likely to be meaningful and which will require special activities to ensure that they become usable parts of the students' accumulated experience.

ACTIVITY

Make a list of the strategies you could use in your teaching to help students process and incorporate information or skills into a form which has meaning for them and which will be retained for future application.

FEEDBACK

There are probably many more ways to achieve meaningful learning than the ones listed below; however, these should be feasible in most teaching contexts.

- Provide a pretest of knowledge, skills or attitudes to give both you and the students an idea of their existing position in relation to the learning to be undertaken.
- Suggest reading assignments before class so that all students have at least thought about the issues to be discussed and perhaps related them to things they already know or problems they have already encountered.

- Introduce topics at a level which you can be sure is understood by everybody; use familiar examples to introduce unfamiliar concepts, e.g. the analogy between the heart and a mechanical pump, or the knee joint and a hinge.
- Use materials, case histories, discussion topics, role plays, etc., to which students can relate on a personal basis. Most students have some experience of illness among their own families and friends and can draw on these experiences to approach clinical problems even at a very early stage in their training.
- Provide alternative learning methods such as self-instructional materials or handouts instead of, or in addition to, traditional methods. The provision of alternative resources and methods which suit different learning styles and preferences helps to improve student performance (Biggs and Telfer, 1983).
- Ensure that group activities have sufficient built-in flexibility to accommodate the needs of the individuals in the group as well as sufficient structure to encourage task completion.
- Consult with students in the setting of objectives for their learning. This option is perhaps more feasible in areas of the course which are not considered to be core, e.g. elective terms, practicum experiences or group assignments. This type of approach ('contracting' – Knowles, 1975), in which the learning objectives and criteria for satisfactory performance are determined jointly by teachers and students, is commonly used in nursing courses (Sasmor, 1984). Contracting provides valuable opportunities for the development of personal strategies for structuring learning and the capacity for self-evaluation.
- Encourage a self-corrective reflexive approach to learning (Mezirow, 1983) that takes an enquiring approach to the process as well as the content of learning. Discussion of the processes by which students arrived at an answer to a question, a solution to a problem or a plan for management makes learning strategies explicit and gives students a chance to compare their personal strategies with their teachers' and colleagues' strategies and, where appropriate, to develop more efficient and effective approaches.
- Actively discourage rote memorization of facts and lists. Set examinations that test understanding and the ability to apply knowledge.
- Plan your teaching to include as much active participation by students as possible. Only by working on and with new knowledge will they be able to make it their own knowledge.

CONDITIONS IN THE LEARNING CONTEXT

ACTIVITY

Drawing on your experience as a learner and teacher, identify the major factors within the learning context or environment that influence learning.

FEEDBACK

The learning context can be defined as those factors which affect the attitudes of your students to each other, to you, your subject and to learning itself. They are difficult factors to define and their exact nature will differ very much from culture to culture, but they can be broadly divided into physical aspects of the environment and psychological or emotional aspects of the environment.

Do your students enjoy learning? Are they interested to learn and motivated to study because of that interest rather than the threat of examinations? Do they co-operate with each other? Do they feel free to approach you for help and to discuss their learning problems with you? Do they feel safe to discuss emotional matters and attitudes with their fellow students? Are they receiving the individual attention that some may need more than others? Are you aware of some of their individual needs and how to help them?

Attitudes to education have changed over the years, under the influence of philosophies held by people like Maslow (1943), Rogers (1969) and Bruner (1962), who stressed the personal development aspects of education and who advocated that conditions should be created which allow students sufficient 'freedom to learn' unhindered by rigid conceptions of the learning task as an information transfer exercise. Dewey (1917) had expressed similar ideas much earlier and more recent and radical approaches have been taken by Illich (1971) and Freire (1970). All are based on the philosophy that people have a natural desire to learn and will undertake learning in the pursuit of personal competence, self-esteem, self-actualization and enjoyment. Knowles (1975) has applied the same principles to the study of adult learning in particular and has concluded that adults are motivated to learn in order to solve problems that have personal relevance for them. All these educators have criticized aspects of traditional education which stress external rewards for learning and which leave little room for creativity and personal development alongside the achievement of set learning objectives.

More traditional views of learning held that students were in nursing school to learn, not to enjoy themselves or to express their individuality. In contrast, modern theories about learning suggest that an investment in the emotional well-being of students will pay off in the form of more positive attitudes towards learning, and ultimately towards nursing responsibilities. Planning for appropriate learning conditions cannot bring about learning if students are not motivated to learn or not courageous enough to seek help with their problems. Admittedly this approach comes more naturally to some teachers than others and many good teachers have always been aware of the importance of the learning context and have developed personal ways of creating it. Orton (1983) carried out research into the learning climate in wards and concluded that 'good learning environments can be identified as those displaying teamwork, good communication and a concern for individual students and their learning needs'.

ACTIVITY

You will have developed some ways of creating a comfortable and productive learning context in your classroom – in other words, you will be aware of certain actions that you take which help both you and your students to work with the subject matter in a way that makes learning effective.

Write down some of the methods that you use. Include physical factors as well as social or psychological ones.

FEEDBACK

Physical factors

Under physical factors you may have listed the following:

- Adequate lighting, ventilation, seating and temperature control.
- Seating arrangements – flexibility in seating arrangements allows for the creation of environments to suit specific learning contexts, for example, students seated in a circle find it easier and more comfortable to have a discussion. If you wish to join the discussion

you should join the circle. Seating arrangements that place you at the front of the class ensure that you do all of the talking. Of course that might be desirable for some contexts but probably not for all.

- Learning materials and resources – these increase the flexibility of classroom activity and allow a variety of approaches to learning with the teacher playing a greater or lesser role as appropriate.
- Sufficient learning spaces to allow students to pursue private study or group activities in relative comfort and close proximity to any necessary resources.
- Convenient and frequent access to hospitals or other institutions in which practical training is occurring. Easy access and allocation of a student common room increases students' feeling of belonging in the institution and contributing to its function.

Social factors

Under social or psychological factors you may have listed the following:

- Your own personality – Most of us have to operate with the personality we have because it is difficult and may not be desirable to change. However, any teacher should be able to create warmth in interaction with a class – this can be done, for example, by avoiding insulting or sarcastic remarks. Walking among students in class or sitting with them will decrease your distance from them and give the impression of approachability.
- Maintaining a working atmosphere in the class is important but there is room for some relaxation to allow for questions, discussion and minor diversions from the topic to explore an unexpected outcome of the lesson. If this type of behaviour is accepted by students and teachers then students are encouraged to think more about the topic and to gain confidence in their own abilities.
- Treating students as individuals may be difficult with a large class but it should be attempted whenever possible. Learning students' names, taking time to praise work well done or to assist with work poorly done will increase the students' motivation to work well and will also provide them with a model to follow when they are teachers themselves.
- Avoiding harsh criticism helps to create trust and students feel more prepared to risk making comments that they want to try out with the teacher and class. It is true that this is sometimes difficult: teachers are only human and students sometimes disappoint them badly. However, while students certainly need to be told when they are wrong or when they are behaving in an undesirable manner,

such criticism should be constructive rather than destructive. Point out what they have done wrong and how they should do it correctly, but try to avoid personal insults such as accusations of stupidity.

- Encouraging students to develop internal standards by which to judge their own efforts increases their level of internal motivation and personal and professional development. Ask for their opinion of their work before you offer yours. Discuss their goals with them and offer constructive feedback on their appropriateness.

- Setting goals with students which are co-operative or individualistic rather than competitive. Johnson and Johnson (1974) have described these three goal structures in education. The competitive goal structure which predominates in traditional educational practice evaluates students against the performance of their fellows. Professional nurses, as we have already seen, need to be able to develop internal goals and standards and to achieve mastery in specific responsibilities – this requires individualistic goal structures in which students are assessed against their achievement of personal goals determined on the basis of individual needs. On the other hand, nurses will work as part of a health-care team and should be familiar with working within co-operative goal structures, where individuals are assessed on the basis of their contribution to the tasks of their group

- Being aware of the process of professional socialization (Smythe, 1984). Simpson (1979), in her classic study of nursing socialization, defined the dimensions of socialization as cognitive preparation to perform the role, orientations to the demands of the role and the appropriate behaviour to meet those demands, and motivation to make the transition from training to work. Opportunities to work alongside practising nurses and acceptance by them as junior colleagues are important to the development of the students' concepts of themselves as nurses. Care should be taken to ensure that the practices and principles taught in the school or classroom are relevant to the realities of practice and either reinforce professional values displayed in practice or explicitly prepare students for divergent value orientations that they might encounter in different environments. Simpson concluded that entering students endorsed views that fitted well with the conception of the ideal nurse that the school wanted to prepare but that the process of their education shifted their views towards a bureaucratic conception of nursing, ideally opposed by the faculty. The curriculum and student assignments on wards emphasized technical, task-oriented nursing and students developed orientations consistent with this emphasis. The implication is that students conform to the real demands made upon them rather than to abstract ideals presented or rehearsed in theoretical contexts (Kramer, 1974, 1985).

This list is by no means complete; however, most of the factors mentioned will be relevant at some time or another in your classes. Some methods may work for you, others may not. You could experiment with those suggestions that appeal to you and see whether they do work within your context.

CONDITIONS WITHIN THE SUBJECT MATTER

Special characteristics of specific subjects or disciplines will demand different skills and abilities of both learners and teachers so, once again, we will not be providing hard and fast rules for creating appropriate conditions, but rather general principles which you can apply when appropriate.

ACTIVITY

Consider the discipline or subject that you teach. Can you represent the key features of that discipline and their relationships to each other in diagrammatic form? What types of learning are required of your students in order to master your subject?

FEEDBACK

If you were able to draw a diagram representing the basic structure of your subject you will now have before you a 'concept map' of your subject. Concept mapping has been described by Novak and Gowin (1984) as a means of helping students to come to grips with the structure of topics they have to learn; it can also be used in assessment of student learning. Smith (1992) applied the cognitive strategies of Novak and Gowin's concept mapping and Vee heuristics to teaching nursing. The aim was to integrate theory and practice. Smith (p 16) reports that students using the Novak and Gowin method rather than traditional modes 'were significantly better able to identify scientific principles to describe why specific steps of a nursing skill were done'.

Perhaps more importantly you can use concept mapping to help you plan your teaching – if you have trouble making connections between key features of your subject, imagine how difficult it will be for your students. Not only must students create their own networks for relating new topics to each other and to existing knowledge but most disciplines will also require learners to undertake a variety of types of learning. Gagne (1976, ch 3) has classified the main outcomes of learning as:

- **verbal information** – the basic store of facts and propositions;
- **intellectual skills** – consisting of the ability to discriminate between stimuli, to develop concepts that organize knowledge and enable the learner to identify a class of objects, and to learn rules which enable the learner to respond to concepts with appropriate actions; these intellectual skills build on each other in the sense that the simpler ones are prerequisites for the more complex;
- **cognitive strategies** – govern the learner's behaviour in dealing with the environment: the learner uses cognitive strategies to think about learning and to solve problems; as we have discussed earlier in this chapter, cognitive strategies may be innate characteristics of the individual but they are also able to be learned and some educators have advocated their importance as educational goals in helping students 'learn how to learn' or 'learn to think' (Bruner, 1962);
- **attitudes** – a system of preferences which affect performance;
- **motor skills** – those manual or technical performances required in the application of what has been learned.

Using this classification you should reconsider the concept map of your subject and identify the various types of learning involved. Do they correspond with the types of learning you had originally identified? Have a close look at any discrepancies and make sure that you can apply the concepts presented to your subject area. It is probable that the emphasis may fall more heavily on some learning outcomes than others but it is also probable that all types of outcomes will be represented in your subject – at least to some extent.

Most learning theories acknowledge these different learning outcomes, although emphasis differs and the strategies advocated for the achievement of each may also differ according to the philosophy and theoretical orientation of the educator. Some stress the sequential approach, in which basic learning outcomes act as prerequisite building blocks for subsequent learning outcomes; for example, children cannot learn to read until they can recognize and discriminate letters of the alphabet. Others see learning as a more idiosyncratic event in which learners incorporate knowledge and skills into existing cognitive structures in a sequence which is relevant to the task at hand, something like fitting pieces into a jigsaw puzzle and gradually building up a complete picture. Mezirow (1983) draws attention to Albert Camus's definition of an intellectual as 'a mind that watches itself', and notes that it also describes how adults learn when they are using critical reflectivity. In fact all of these learning strategies are likely to be appropriate at different stages and in different contexts. The teacher's task is to ensure that students are sufficiently flexible to employ the most appropriate strategy for the learning objectives.

Problem-based learning and attention to the processes of learning that encourage active student involvement and application of learned knowledge and skills to novel situations are methods for increasing students' intellectual flexibility (Boud and Feletti, 1991). Failure to promote this flexibility in students results in the all too familiar situation in which students learn facts, discriminations, concepts and principles which are stored in memory in a way that allows retrieval for examination purposes but which does not facilitate transfer to the practical situation. The problem is analogous to a filing system which is arranged according to date of receipt rather than function of documents. Retrieval of documents stored in the month of March is simple, as is recall of definitions learned in physiology lectures; however retrieval of documents required for the solution of a specific business problem will require a good deal of inefficient searching and trial and error, as would the solution of a clinical problem presenting as physiological disturbance. Knowledge which is not stored as part of a functional cognitive structure will not be efficiently used.

ACTIVITY

Refer to the first activity in this chapter, in which you identified a personal learning experience which was either effective or ineffective. From your analysis of the reasons for the effectiveness of that experience and from your reading of this chapter work out some principles that describe the necessary conditions for learning knowledge, attitudes and skills.

FEEDBACK

Once again there are no right or wrong answers in this activity. Conditions for learning will vary a great deal among cultures and teaching situations; however, in general the following principles apply.

CONDITIONS FOR LEARNING KNOWLEDGE

For simplicity we will include Gagne's verbal information, intellectual skills and cognitive strategies under the general heading of 'knowledge'. Knowledge is made up of the facts of the subject and the learners' ability to use those facts to think and solve problems.

- Students must be presented with information in a form that they can understand. The most obvious example is that students must be familiar with the vocabulary and the concepts used. This is a common problem in nursing courses, where many technical terms are needed. At a different level students must understand why they have to learn that information and how it can be made to fit with what they already know. In other words, the information must be relevant to them.
- Students must be able to store information in a way that facilitates its functional retrieval. If students are presented with information which is totally unfamiliar they may be unable to relate it to existing knowledge or to future tasks, they will need advance organizers to help them classify the new information and they will need practical tasks to encourage them to use the new information so that it forms part of a usable cognitive framework. Your own 'concept map' of the subject might help you to make functional connections explicit for the students. Helping students to classify new information simplifies the learning task because students can include the new information under more general principles which are already known, with the result that only specific details need to be learned. For example, if we classify a drug as belonging to the category of beta-blockers then students who know about the general characteristics of beta-blockers will need to learn only those details, such as toxicity levels, which are specific to that particular drug.
- Students must be able to use the information they have learned to perform tasks or to solve problems. Unless students are given practice in using the information they have learned it will be quickly forgotten. To ensure that transfer to clinical nursing is achieved it is important that the opportunity for practice occurs in situations as close as possible to situations they will encounter in reality (see simulations in Chapter 5). But it isn't enough that we teach students to solve a particular type of problem using particular sets of information. Health-care problems are not predictable, patients will present with problems which are difficult to classify, traditional therapies may fail. No training course can ever hope to cover all the possible situations the nurse will confront. Students should

therefore be encouraged to strengthen and develop cognitive strategies that will enable them to think on the job, to create innovative solutions to unusual problems and to generalize their professional and personal experiences to responsive nursing practice. Remember that there are individual differences in students' preferred cognitive strategies and in their aptitudes for learning different types of information. Some students may need more time, assistance and remedial work than others to achieve similar levels of competence.

- Students must have knowledge of the effectiveness of their use of information. Feedback on the effectiveness of the cognitive strategies students use is essential if students are to maximize their potential. Feedback should be specific and diagnostic to enable students to rectify specific learning problems. It is not sufficient to say that the students' patient management plan is wrong, you must go through it with her/him and discuss both its strong points and its weak points to guide the student's processes of problem analysis. Discussions of process as well as content should be an integral part of learning, as should be exercises in which students are able to judge their own performance and develop internal standards which are professionally appropriate.

CONDITIONS FOR LEARNING ATTITUDES

Attitudes may be defined as feelings, beliefs, values or preferences that influence the way the student behaves.

- Students cannot be taught attitudes in the same way that they are taught information or skills. Because attitudes are involved with emotions they are personal and less accessible to the teacher. For this reason they are also difficult to assess; sources of external motivation are rarely effective in shaping desirable attitudes. It is highly desirable that nurses should have some particular attitudes which will assist them to gain the co-operation and trust of their patients and which will ensure that they conduct their professional tasks with responsibility. Teachers must therefore provide conditions in which favourable attitudes can develop. It is not sufficient to leave attitude formation to chance since students may well be exposed to quite powerful experiences which predispose to the formation of attitudes that are not desired learning outcomes (see Simpson, 1979).
- Students must be helped to recognize their existing attitudes. Students come to nursing school with preconceived ideas about the

role of a nurse, the causes of illness, the feelings of patients, and many other aspects of health care. These ideas will be the products of their previous experiences and education. Some may be congruent with nursing practice and some may not. Before the incongruent attitudes can be changed the students must recognize them. Recognition of existing attitudes can be encouraged by discussion of controversial issues in class or by setting up activities in which students play roles (see Chapter 4).

- Students should be provided with new information which will challenge existing attitudes. For example, as students come to know more about the physiology of certain diseases they may feel less worried about helping people with those diseases; as they become more skilled at specific tasks they may become less reticent about direct patient contact, as they become more familiar with nursing roles they may correct previous inaccurate perceptions.

- Students should be given the opportunity to test new attitudes. Feedback is as important in the development of new attitudes as it is in the learning of knowledge or skills. For example, a student may observe that a nurse who has a respectful attitude towards elderly patients is better able to gain their co-operation. Opportunities for work with elderly patients will then enable the student to try out aspects of behaviour that were observed. It is important to expose students to as many models of desired behaviour as possible. Opportunities for practice of modelled behaviour may be provided by role play or class discussion prior to actual clinical contact but in all circumstances feedback is important so that the student realizes how his or her attitudes influenced performance. Ideally, observation of videotape replay provides the most graphic feedback to students of their attitudes and behaviour.

CONDITIONS FOR LEARNING SKILLS

Skills are performances that students learn through practice. In most cases they will be manual skills, such as giving an injection or taking a blood pressure, but they may also be skills which involve communication, e.g. talking with a patient to explain a procedure.

- Students must know what it is they are expected to be able to do. Students must observe someone demonstrating the skill effectively. Sometimes films are used to demonstrate skills which are difficult to set up in the classroom.

- Students must know how the skill is performed. Most skills have a number of component subskills within them, each of which must be mastered before the student can perform the total skill. Each component subskill must therefore be demonstrated specifically so that the students' attention is drawn to specific aspects which contribute to effective performance. For example, adequate hand-washing is a necessary component skill in applying a sterile dressing.

- Students must practise the skill. Knowing how to perform the skill is not sufficient. There is a big difference between knowing how and actually doing well. In many cases practice may be difficult to obtain because it may involve risk or discomfort to patients. In such cases it is important to provide students with the opportunity to practise in a situation which resembles the real one closely but which does not carry any risks. This type of exercise is called a simulation. One example is the use of an orange to teach students how to give an injection. Another is for students to practise procedures on one another before they try them on people who are ill. As students begin to master the skill they may be progressively moved from simulation classes to real settings such as clinics. Practice in the real situation must be supervised until the teacher is confident that the skill has been mastered. Individual differences in aptitudes among students mean that students will not all achieve mastery at the same rate and flexibility should be built in to allow for longer practice periods and more feedback for those students who require it. It is unrealistic to assume that all will be equally skilled at the end of a course unless steps have been taken to diagnose those with a difficulty and provide remedial instruction.
- Students must receive feedback on their performance. Practice alone is not sufficient for mastery of a skill: practice must be accompanied by knowledge of whether the performance is satisfactory. Feedback may be given by the teacher, fellow students, patients or students themselves. Feedback must be specific and diagnostic – it must help the student identify specific aspects of performance that require further work. The ultimate aim of skill learning should be to transfer the students' dependence from the teacher's evaluation to personal or self-evaluation.

SUMMARY

Helping students learn is the primary role of the teacher. This chapter has examined some of the factors within the student, the learning context and the subject matter which influence student learning. Feasible strategies are available for the teacher to employ in each of those areas; all such strategies depend on the teacher's willingness to become personally involved with students. Getting to know students' individual characteristics and needs, creating a climate of trust in which students can develop professional self-image and personal self-esteem, creating learning experiences which motivate, which allow for individual differences, active involvement, transfer and generalization of learned information and skills, providing specific constructive feedback and encouraging growing self-reliance are essential parts of a nurse educator's role. The following chapters provide specific suggestions for creating those conditions in the variety of learning contexts found in schools of nursing.

Managing the learning session

4

INTRODUCTION

This chapter deals with the practical aspects of managing the learning session. In the previous chapters we have dealt with how you would decide what to teach and how you would decide which teaching methods to use. In this chapter we will look in more detail at some of those methods.

When you have finished this chapter you should be able to manage the following teaching methods effectively:

- lectures;
- small-group discussions;
- role play and other simulations;
- critical incidents and other reflective activities, such as journalling;
- independent learning.

Clinical teaching is dealt with in the following chapter.

In your use of all of these methods, remember the conditions for learning discussed in Chapter 3. Your task as teacher is to try to create those conditions by skilful use of the methods described in this chapter. These methods have been chosen because they are the methods most commonly used by nurse teachers. You may already be familiar with, and skilled in, the use of some of the methods and you may wish to try integrating different aspects of the methods to increase the students' involvement with, and understanding of, what they need to learn. The references quoted in this chapter provide many interesting suggestions for innovations in teaching.

Many teachers have found they need a repertoire of teaching skills to use as they lecture, facilitate group discussion, and in fact during any teaching method where the aim is to encourage students to learn. We have mentioned elsewhere (Chapters 2 and 3) the importance of the relevance of the learning sessions, the need to integrate theory with practice and the approach to learning the students bring to the session. Your selection of learning activities will depend on a good 'fit' between the subject matter, its practical application and an appreciation of the perspective your students have on the material you will be presenting.

HOW WILL YOU DECIDE WHAT LEARNING ACTIVITIES TO USE?

ACTIVITY

The following criteria, taken from Crotty (1989), may be helpful in selecting learning activities for your students. Which criteria would you consider using to help you choose learning activities for your students? What would influence your choice?

Does the learning activity:

- allow students to make an informed choice regarding the type of learning activity they engage in and to reflect on the consequences of their choice?
- encourage students to participate in the learning experience?
- require students to enquire into nursing practices and procedures and the application of research to them?
- involve students in interaction and experience with students?
- engage students in applying a known nursing concept to a different nursing setting?
- require students to examine health-care problems within a broader economic and social context?
- involve students in applying nursing theory to practice?
- give students the opportunity of working with others in a team?
- engage students in the analysis and solving of a problem?
- appear to be relevant to students' learning needs?
- encourage students to accept responsibility for their own learning?

(Source: adapted from Crotty, 1989)

FEEDBACK

First of all, you have probably chosen the criteria that centre on encouraging students to participate, to interact with patients, to work with others in a team, and to accept responsibility for their own learning relevant to their learning needs, in other words, the well known and accepted teaching and learning criteria. You may have found some of the others interesting, as they give importance to selecting a learning experience which involves students in critical thinking and questioning about the research base of nursing practices, the appropriateness of some nursing concepts for some settings and the need to consider nursing in a wider economic and social context.

So the learning activities you use do more than simply introduce variety to keep students active and involved. They can lead to a deeper understanding of the students' own capacity for learning and their ability to apply their knowledge effectively. It is a good idea to keep these criteria in mind as you work your way through the teaching methods that follow. Later in the chapter we will pursue how learning activities can be developed within the established teaching methods.

THE LECTURE

PLANNING A LECTURE

Lectures are most useful when they are used to provide students with an overview of what they must know in a particular topic area. Lectures are best used to convey information which explains the relationships between detailed concepts in the topic, and which is not readily available elsewhere.

ACTIVITY

1. Select a topic about which you would normally give a lecture.
2. Write down a list of objectives for that lecture in terms of what you hope your students will gain from it.
3. List the key concepts or ideas which would form the main content of the lecture.
4. Plan the structure of your lecture, perhaps using a diagram to show the relationships between your key concepts, the sequence in which you will present them and the main examples you will use to expand your ideas.
5. Describe the teaching aids or resources you would use to help you make the lecture effective.
6. How will you check whether your objectives have been achieved?

FEEDBACK

Feedback for this activity will be arranged according to each of those tasks you have done in planning your lecture.

Selection of a topic

Look at your topic again. Is your lecture the only formal teaching students will receive on that topic? Are the textbooks up to date in that area and are they easy for your students to understand? Is the topic one that has components of skills and attitudes as well as the knowledge you will be presenting in the lecture? Is the topic one with which your students usually have difficulty or is it fairly straightforward? Is the topic one that generates a lot of student interest or do they usually find it dull or uninteresting?

Objectives for the lecture

Your answers to the questions about your topic should help you to decide what your objectives for the lecture are. For example, if the topic is one which is not well covered by textbooks or other areas of teaching such as tutorials or clinical experiences your main objectives for the lecture may include the intention that students should be able to take a set of lecture notes which can serve as accurate reference material for their future learning (information lecture).

If the topic is one which students usually find difficult to understand your objectives may include the intention that students will derive from the lecture a clearer picture of the main concepts and ideas and their relationships and thus develop a mental structure into which they can fit some of the more detailed aspects of the topic they will read about in their textbooks (explanation lecture).

If the lecture is part of a larger set of experiences which include opportunities for learning skills and attitudes related to the topic, your objectives might be concerned with students gaining an overview of the topic and the relative importance of its component parts (overview lecture).

If the topic is one which students usually find dull the objectives of the lecture should be concerned with students' motivation to learn the topic (motivation lecture).

For convenience of reference each of these lectures has been given a name which appears in brackets at the end of the description. Of course, many lectures will contain elements of all or most of those objectives, but it is important nevertheless to decide what your objectives are so that you can plan a style and sequence of presentation that will be most effective in achieving them.

Content of the lecture

Look at the key ideas and concepts you have decided to include in your lecture. Are they appropriate for your objectives? Do they motivate the student to want to learn the topic? Do they provide information which is not covered elsewhere or are they unnecessarily detailed, repeating essentially what is in the textbooks? Do they explain and put into context the relationship of the content of this lecture to the rest of the course?

Structure of the lecture

Bligh (1972), Brown (1978), Lowman (1984) and Brookfield (1991) have all described a variety of lecture structures which may be used. Broadly, lectures fall into two main structure types, classical and problem-centred. The classical structure proceeds logically through information which is (usually) ordered from simple to complex, from normal to abnormal, from general principles to specific examples, leading the student progressively to an understanding of the overall topic through knowledge of its parts. The problem-centred structure seems, at times, to do just the opposite, often providing examples of complex problems as the starting point and progressing through analysis of general principles, basic mechanisms and explanatory simpler information.

The structure you choose should depend on your personal preferences and on the objectives of the lecture. Teachers are usually more comfortable with the classical structure because it resembles the traditional explanatory structure of most disciplines and is the structure with which most teachers are familiar. It is also an easier structure for students to follow if their purpose is to take comprehensive notes from the lecture (information lecture). The problem-centred structure, on the other hand, is a useful strategy for those lectures that are seen by students to be dull or even irrelevant (motivation lecture). By providing clinical nursing problems as the basis for the information to be transmitted, the teacher helps the students to see why this information is necessary and how it fits into the job they are being trained for. Since the problem-centred lecture usually starts with a question it should also stimulate students' curiosity to follow the lecture through and arrive at the answer. A well planned problem-centred lecture can aid students to understand difficult concepts and their relationships to each other in a context which is seen to be pertinent to the students' future role (explanation lecture, overview lecture). Problem-centred lectures, however, often result in less comprehensive students' notes since the emphasis is on the process of relating ideas to problems and solutions rather than on presenting a systematic body of information. Whichever structure you have chosen, the general principles for presentation of the lecture apply.

- Always start with a brief description of what you intend to cover and the general structure you intend to follow. Remind students of related information that they already know and of the reasons why the topic of this lecture is important for them. Students are more motivated to learn when they know what they are expected to learn and why they need to learn it. Reminding students of relevant previous learning helps them to grasp the meaning of new information more easily.
- Use a series of major headings or subheadings on the board or in student handouts to signpost the direction in which you are heading and to ensure that students can organize their thinking and their note-taking.
- Use special techniques to emphasize the most important points in the lecture. There are a number of ways to do this.
  - You can write key words or phrases on the chalkboard.
  - You can use audiovisual aids.
  - You can change the volume or expression of your voice to awaken students' attention.
  - You can repeat the important points for emphasis.
  - You can pause to ask the class a question about the important points.
  - You can use specific phrases to draw attention, such as 'make sure you understand this'.
- Summarize periodically the information you have covered. This enables students to review what you have said and to ensure that they are following your line of evidence or information.
- Encourage students to be actively involved during the lecture; for example, give them a problem to solve or a question to answer. Active involvement serves two purposes:
  - Students remember information better if they have to think about it as well as just copy it into their notes.
  - Research has shown that most students lose concentration, and their attention to the lecture starts to decrease after about 15–20 minutes (Bligh, 1972, p 73); providing some activity after 20

minutes of the lecture serves to wake students up and to catch their attention again.

(Some more ways of encouraging active participation in the lecture will be discussed in a following section).

- End the lecture by repeating the main points covered and by telling the students what the next lecture or teaching session will cover. It is often stimulating to end the lecture by raising the most contentious and unresolved issues from the lecture because it creates a future-oriented inquiry state of mind and encourages students to investigate some of the issues (Brookfield, 1991).

Teaching aids and resources

Your objectives for the lecture should also guide you in deciding what teaching aids and resources you want to use. Handouts are a useful resource in 'information' lectures because they relieve the student of some of the burden of note-taking. Handouts may provide full information or an outline of headings or main points. If your lecture is predominantly an 'explanation' lecture you may wish to use a number of diagrams. Some teachers prefer to draw diagrams on the chalkboard as they go along but others find that prepared overhead transparencies allow time to be saved and ensure the clarity of the diagram. Diagrams can also be provided as handouts to avoid transcription errors, which often result from hurried copying by students. Modern computer audiovisual resources make it possible to project diagrams stored on your own computer discs. If your lecture is an 'overview' lecture or a 'motivation' lecture you may find that the use of colour photographs, motion pictures or videocassettes helps you to demonstrate aspects of the nurse's role which are difficult to describe but which explain the importance of the topic to be learned or demonstrate its skill and attitudinal components.

Check on achievement of objectives

If you are an experienced lecturer, you may be able to tell from audience non-verbal reaction whether your students are keeping up with the lecture or whether they have drifted off. Besides looking for informal cues such as an increase in the level of background conversation, a cessation of note-taking or an increased incidence of puzzled faces you can also arrange for formal gathering of feedback on students' understanding. You may leave time for questions during or after the lecture (particularly if your class is a small one). You may wish to ask students to fill out forms which provide feedback on specific aspects of your lecturing technique; you may rely on spot tests of lecture content in tutorials or, in the long term, you may check performance on your lecture topics (in formal examinations). One useful method is to schedule follow-up tutorials on specific key points from the lecture and to invite students to attend for the purpose of clarifying their understanding. Such tutorials help both the teacher and the students to identify problem areas in teaching and learning.

You may wish to undertake the following activity, which provides practice in applying these principles of lecture planning.

ACTIVITY

Choose another topic about which you may be asked to give a lecture. Write a lecture outline for that topic following the guidelines suggested in the previous activity. Remember to define your objectives, outline your content, map out your structure and plan the resources and feedback mechanisms you will use.

FEEDBACK

Feedback for this activity is a lecture outline using contraceptive methods as an example topic.

LECTURE OUTLINE

- **Topic**: Contraceptive methods
- **Learners**: Community Health Nurses
- **Purpose**: The lecture is intended to provide an overview of the topic, since a comprehensive and accurate account of the topic is provided in the textbook.
- **Objectives**: After attending the lecture nurses should be able to describe the mechanism of action of the four main types of contraceptive, and explain the indications and contraindications for each that contribute to choice of method.

Content, structure and resources

- **Introduction:**
State and clarify the objectives for the lecture.

Describe the nurse's future likely role in advising about contraception.

Recall previous learning by asking nurses to write down a classification of the ways in which conception might be prevented.

- **Key points:**
1. Conception may be prevented by preventing ovulation, fertilization or implantation (*resource*: overhead transparency diagram of sites of action of main contraceptives).
2. Prevention of ovulation (*resource*: handouts with graphs of ovulatory cycle – ask nurses to label graph curves with appropriate hormones). Describe mechanisms of action of hormonal contraceptives and the advantages and disadvantages.

(Stop for questions.)

3. Prevention of fertilization – describe rhythm method (*resource*: handout of graph of ovulatory cycle).

(Stop for discussion of advantages and disadvantages of rhythm method.)

Describe barrier methods, how they work and advantages and disadvantages (*resources*: samples and/or diagrams).

(Summarize main points and allow a few minutes for questions.)

4. Prevention of implantation – intrauterine devices – how they work, who they are suitable for (*resources*: samples and diagrams).

- **Clinical problem:**
Present a brief case history and ask students to form small groups with those in adjacent seats to decide on the most appropriate contraceptive to recommend.

Obtain responses from two or three groups.

Provide feedback to class on the correct choice and the reason for it. Use this feedback to summarize the main points covered in the lecture.

- **Closure:**
Tutorial to follow this lecture will deal with questions arising from the lecture. Advise students to read relevant chapters in the textbook.

Outline of handout to be used in lecture

1. Objectives for the lecture
2. Use the following questions as headings with space for students' notes:

    (a) How do the hormonal contraceptives work?

(b) What is the basis of the rhythm method?
(c) What are the most reliable barrier contraceptives?
(d) What are the main indications for the use of IUD?
3.   Graph of ovulatory cycle – labelling to be completed by students
4.   Summary list of main contraindications to use of each of the contraceptives described.

Summary

Your lecture outline may be quite different from the one suggested here. That does not matter; the important thing is to remember the basic principles:

- **Introduction**:
  To set objectives
  To motivate
  To remind them of other related knowledge
- **Logical organization**:
  Use lists of key points, handouts
- **Emphasize main points**:
  Use audiovisual aids, questions, repetition
- **Student participation**:
  Buzz groups, question time, incomplete handouts
- **Summarize**:
  At the end of each section
  At the end of the lecture
- **Closure**:
  Refer to other classes plus follow-up activities
  Check their understanding.

Presenting a lecture

Of course, knowing how to plan a lecture is only half of the story. Even a well planned lecture will suffer from poor presentation by the lecturer. Skills in presentation can only be gained by practice and feedback on performance. We will be dealing with evaluation of teaching skills in a later chapter, but in the meantime you might like to consider some informal ways of seeking feedback on your lecturing skills. You could, if you have the resources, request that your lectures be videotaped so that you can get a student's eye view of yourself, or if that is not possible you may make an audiotape of your lectures so that you can at least hear what your lecture sounded like. This is an excellent way of finding out how well you have structured your presentation and your explanations. Another option is to develop a reciprocal arrangement with a trusted fellow teacher who can observe your lectures and also be observed by you for the purposes of constructive suggestions for improvement. Start by asking for feedback on areas of your teaching that concern you and gradually build up to those areas such as personal mannerisms, which may be more personally threatening.

As you become more comfortable with some of the basic suggestions presented in this book you may wish to experiment with different methods of involving students or with different ways of presenting material or using audiovisual aids. Many helpful suggestions can be found in Bligh, 1972; Powell, 1973; Brown, 1978; Ericksen, 1984; Eble, 1988; Brookfield, 1991; and Quinn, 1994.

SMALL-GROUP DISCUSSION

In this section of the chapter we will be looking at small groups used as a method for increasing student discussion. For our purposes a small group will be defined as a group of less than 15 people who are meeting for an educational purpose. There are many different ways in which learning in small groups may be encouraged. The way that you plan and conduct small-group learning should be determined by two considerations:

- what you are trying to achieve – your objectives for the session;
- what you and your students are comfortable with.

Many teachers complain that their students will not participate in group discussion so that teachers might just as well give a lecture to a large group. The following activities and suggestions are intended to help you overcome this problem and to develop ways for gaining maximum benefit from small-group learning sessions.

The first consideration is to decide for what purposes small-group learning is best suited.

ACTIVITY

What types of learning can be achieved more effectively in small groups than in other ways? Make a list of the teaching situations in which you would choose to use a small group rather than another type of learning situation.

FEEDBACK

Small-group sessions are useful for:

- involving students as active participants in the learning task, rather than as passive listeners;
- developing skills in teamwork and co-operation;
- developing manual, physical or communication skills through practice and feedback from the teacher and other students;
- providing practice in applying knowledge to solving problems individually or as a member of a group;
- encouraging students to try out new attitudes and ideas with a group of their peers;
- providing opportunities for students to have close contact with a teacher and check out their understanding.

You may also have thought of other purposes, but if you found it difficult to answer the questions in this activity you should refer back to Chapter 3. The important thing to remember about the purposes of small-group learning is that the interaction among members of the group is the critical event. Learning how to approach and solve problems, developing skills and forming attitudes can be achieved in small groups because the members of the group can help and stimulate each other to work through whatever the learning task is.

The help and support that group members can provide for each other may not be present in the initial stages of group work, but if the teacher is sensitive and able to help this climate of support to develop, then productive, co-operative relationships usually result. In fact, one of the most important purposes of group work is to help students develop skills in teamwork. Such skills will be important in the performance of their clinical tasks.

PHYSICAL ENVIRONMENT

Small-group function is facilitated by an environment that allows a degree of relaxation by participants. If it is possible to provide comfortable chairs, tea- or coffee-making facilities and pleasant, private surroundings – so much the better. Most teachers, however, will have to make do with standard teaching accommodation, but the crucial point to remember is that if you want students to talk to each other then seating must be arranged so that they can comfortably see each other.

The most effective seating arrangement for a discussion group is to have all participants seated so that they are facing each other. Usually this is achieved by placing seats in a circle or an oval. If the group's task will require students to do some writing, a table can be placed in the centre. This sort of arrangement can also be achieved in a traditional science laboratory without too much trouble by arrangement of seats around the end and sides of a laboratory bench. The same effect can also be achieved (although not so comfortably) in an ordinary lecture theatre by asking students to turn sideways in their seats to talk with students in the row behind, or in front. Whenever possible, if you, the teacher, are to take part in the discussion you should be seated in the circle too. If the teacher sits apart from the group, students will automatically assume the role they have in a lecture and expect the teacher to do all the talking – which brings us to a consideration of the role of the teacher in small-group discussion.

ACTIVITY

Next time that you are involved in a group discussion take notice of what is happening in the group. The group you observe may be a learning group or an informal meeting for social or administrative purposes. To help you in your observations of the group you may like to keep the following questions in mind:

- Who spoke first?
- Who seemed to be the 'leader' of the group – what was that person doing which gave you the impression that he or she was the leader?
- Who talked to whom?
- What was the emotional climate in the group like – were people happy, productive, bored, aggressive? What were the factors contributing to that climate?
- Were there any patterns that emerged in the behaviour of the members of the group?
- From your observations of the group can you draw any conclusions about factors that influence the effectiveness of discussion in groups?

FEEDBACK

There are many excellent books available which deal with small-group dynamics in general (e.g. McLeish, 1973; Abercrombie, 1969; Miles, 1981; Jacques, 1984; Goodall, 1990; Schultz, 1989) and in nursing in particular (e.g. Wilson, 1985; Clark, 1987; Quinn, 1994). Some of the main points which bear on the function of small discussion groups are summarized below.

THE ROLE OF THE TEACHER

There are no hard and fast rules for the role the teacher will play in the group. Obviously the teacher's role will vary with the objectives of the discussion and with the types of student who are being taught. The main thing to remember is that it is an inefficient use of time if the members of a small group spend their time listening to what the teacher has to say, because this is in effect a lecture which might just as easily be given to a large group of students. Of course, for some types of learning objective the teacher will have a major role to play, perhaps by demonstrating a particular clinical skill or in guiding students through difficult material towards an understanding of the main concepts. However, even though the teacher has a major role, the key to learning lies in the students' ability to participate in practice of the skill or in thinking through the difficult aspects of a problem. For other types of learning objective it may be more appropriate for the teacher to attempt to be an equal member of the group, allowing other group members to take leadership where appropriate. This approach is most appropriate where the intention is to stimulate students to examine issues, attitudes or feelings in areas in which expertise is less important than personal experience. Depending on the maturity of the group the teacher may find it necessary to play an intermediate role, that of a facilitator – a friendly guide who keeps a watchful eye on the process of the group and intervenes with sensitivity to ensure that objectives are achieved and that a positive climate is maintained in the group.

THE ROLE OF THE STUDENTS

Small-group discussion offers the students the chance to learn by doing. Students must therefore come to the group prepared to work. Since many students' previous educational experiences have accustomed them to a fairly passive approach to learning, students do not always find it easy to adapt to a learning situation in which they must take responsibility for what happens during their time together with the teacher. Sometimes they express impatience with the process of group discussion and insist that they would learn more if the teacher would just tell them what it is that they are supposed to know. In some cases previous bad experiences of small-group learning may have resulted in frustration or withdrawal from participation. Some of these negative reactions to small-group work can be forestalled by the teacher if she/he is aware of the dynamics of group interaction and of approaches that provide structure where necessary and freedom where desirable in order to minimize frustration and maximize satisfaction and productivity.

Experts in the behaviour of people in groups state that all groups go through six broad stages of development. These stages are said to occur in some form regardless of the task of the group, the type of participant or the duration of the group's meeting.

- **Stage 1: Getting to know each other.** In this stage little work is done and group members talk to each other on a fairly superficial level while they become comfortable with each other. The teacher can help students through this stage by creating a warm friendly atmosphere and by inviting students to talk with each other informally before they begin the task.
- **Stage 2: Defining the purpose of the meeting.** In this stage group members attempt to sort out the purpose of the meeting; they sometimes experience a lack of direction or frustration and may become impatient. The teacher can help here by guiding discussion in useful directions or by helping students to clarify what they expect to achieve in the group.
- **Stage 3: Establishing working rules and norms for behaviour.** In this stage ground rules are established. Group members may decide on a strategy for achieving the task, or an order of business to attend to.
- **Stage 4: Active contribution.** By this stage group members have a commitment to the group and its task. Co-operation increases and decisions are made (explicitly or implicitly) about who will do what and when to in order achieve the task.
- **Stage 5: A sense of accomplishment.** Members undertake effective group work to complete their task. At this stage group members may feel pleased with themselves and the mood of the group is usually a positive one.
- **Stage 6: The end of the task.** Group members 'wind down' from the task and carry out final jobs associated with it. The coherence of the group begins to break down.

Of course, some of these stages will assume more prominence than others according to the tasks or objectives of the group. For example, a group meeting for the main purpose of learning how to pass a nasogastric tube will spend most of its time and energy in stages 4 and 5.

On the other hand, a group which has as its objective the development of a nursing plan for a given patient case may need to spend considerable time in stages 2 and 3 before they can hope to be productive in stages 4 and 5. Stage 1 is essential for all groups where the students and the teacher have not worked together before.

Occasionally a group may have more difficulty in one or other stage, particularly in stages 2 and 3. If you are aware that these are normal phases that groups pass through, you will be able to help resolve some of the conflicts so that the group can move on to productive activity. As students become more experienced at working in groups they may also begin to take facilitatory roles in some of the more problematic stages. Since one of the aims of group discussion is to improve students' ability to work together they should be encouraged to understand the processes of the group and to accept responsibility for ensuring its effective function.

When the members of a group work together for a period of time it may also be possible to observe certain roles emerging. You may have noted these roles in your observations of a group. In general the roles fall into two categories – roles associated with the task and roles associated with the social maintenance of the group. Task roles may include initiating action, doing routine chores, gathering information, assigning jobs, drawing group members back to the task, keeping discussion on the track and evaluating group output. Social roles may include keeping interpersonal relations pleasant, handling conflict, providing encouragement, relieving tension through humour, giving silent members a chance to be heard and observing and commenting on the process of the group. All of these roles may of course be filled by the experienced teacher; however, one of the objectives of any small-group learning session should be to encourage students to develop skills in some of those roles themselves, since those skills will be transferable to their professional work on the wards and in the community.

Now that we have considered some of the factors which influence the way learning groups work, it may be useful to turn to a consideration of factors that sometimes impede the function of the group.

ACTIVITY

Think back to the group that you observed or to some other group in which you have recently participated as teacher or learner. What were some of the problems which arose in the process of the group discussion and what could the group facilitator or teacher have done to avoid those problems?

FEEDBACK

Problems for the group leader:

- **Teachers are often tempted to take over the group and do most of the talking or, in the case of skill-learning, to do most of the work.** Students may be willing for this to happen because it saves them from having to work. One of the hardest things for a teacher to learn is to tolerate silence in the learning group. Sometimes a period of silence means that people are thinking and will soon share their thoughts with the rest of the group – if the teacher hurries in to fill the gap the students will not be able to take full advantage of the group activity. Similarly, if the teacher takes up all the available time demonstrating a particular skill students will have no opportunity to do it themselves. Watching is not a substitute for doing.

- **Talkative students may dominate the group, making it difficult for quiet or shy students to enter the discussion.** Teachers must develop tactful ways to control dominant students and encourage quiet students. This may be done by gentle probing such as (to a quiet student): 'What do you think about that?' or 'Is that the way you think it should be done?' A dominant group member can sometimes be given tasks to do which will occupy that person and direct their energy in a productive way. They could, for example, be made responsible for writing the group's findings on the board. Or the teacher can tactfully direct questions elsewhere, for example (to dominant student): 'So that's what you have experienced with this problem in your clinic'; and (to the rest of group): 'Have the rest of you had any other sorts of experience?'

- **Group discussion may become sidetracked from the main purposes of the discussion.** To some extent this may be a good thing. Groups should be able to talk about interesting side issues which crop up. These discussions will also contribute to their learning. However, you will have to judge when the side issues are taking too much time away from the main object of the discussion. You can get the group back on to the track by saying something like: 'That's an interesting point, which we could look at later, but let's get back to the main point and see what we should do about it first'. Sometimes, as the group begins to function better, some of your students may adopt these 'facilitator roles' as well and should be encouraged to do so.

- **The group discussion may become nothing more than a question and answer session where you ask questions or respond to**

students' questions. This is a popular format often seen in small-group sessions after a lecture and it does have a place for clarifying understanding. However it may be time-wasting for some students who are not involved in the discussions. A better way is to ask students for their questions at the beginning and then to set the group the task of answering them. You might act as an extra resource if necessary. Students then benefit not only from having their questions answered but from having to work out and deliver explanations to each other. Explaining is an excellent test and reinforcer of learning.

- **The teacher may not organize the time well enough to allow everyone to benefit from the session.** For example, if the group members are expected to learn a skill the session should be organized so that all members have an opportunity for some practice and feedback on their performance.

- **The discussion may enter areas in which neither the teacher nor the students have the knowledge or skills to proceed productively.** Some teachers find this threatening and tend to direct students towards other more comfortable areas, resulting in the students feeling frustrated and sometimes losing trust or confidence in the teacher. This situation may be avoided by establishing norms or ground rules early in the discussion that clarify your role as a resource for the group rather than as an expert with all of the answers. As a resource you should be able to help the students to determine where they can find the information or skills that are lacking.

In summary, an effective group leader should plan activities which will achieve the learning objectives and encourage student interaction. Productive group discussion cannot be left to 'just happen'. The teacher or group leader and the students must know what the aim of the discussion or activity is and the teacher must be prepared to take action when necessary to create conditions which will be best for the group task. Sometimes this means suggesting an activity, providing information or helping students to overcome personal differences and sometimes it means having the skill, the patience and the trust to leave students to their own devices at the appropriate time.

Some excellent suggestions for maximizing group effectiveness can be found in Smallegan, 1982; Clark, 1987; Lowman, 1984 and Brookfield, 1991. Detailed suggestions for specific activities in specific topics are also provided in subsequent chapters in this book.

PLANNING A SMALL-GROUP SESSION

ACTIVITY

Now that you have some new ideas about making groups work it will be helpful if you put them into practice to see how well they work with your subject and your students. Plan a small-group session for a topic that you teach. Pay particular attention to the following.

- How will you introduce the topic?
- How will you encourage participation by group members?
- How will you finish off the discussion or activity?

FEEDBACK

Needless to say, you should begin your planning by deciding what are the objectives of the learning session. Don't forget that, since you are using a small group for the topic, you should try to include objectives which make use of the capacity for practice, interaction and feedback. In other words you should use the small group as an opportunity for attitudes- and skill-learning as well as the acquisition of knowledge. Since you may not always have complete control over the direction in which students take the discussion you should give careful thought to the key areas or key questions you would like to be addressed by the group. If their discussions take them into those areas, well and good; if not, you can be prepared to judiciously insert probing or leading questions that will bring those key issues to the fore.

Decide on the level of autonomy you wish the group to have and therefore on the level of control you wish to exert over the activities of the group. If you intend to maintain a low profile it will be particularly important for you to provide an introduction to the topic that will allow the students to define its scope and direction without having to guess what you want them to do.

The following suggestions are an incomplete list of strategies you may use for getting the group started and keeping it going.

STARTING THE GROUP DISCUSSION

The way you start the discussion should motivate students to want to talk about the topic or undertake the task.

Use a case study, film or story to focus students on the topic and help them to see its relevance to the tasks of the nurse.

Show enthusiasm for the topic and an interest in tackling the problem or procedure yourself.

Try to choose a problem or task that the students see as important – you might want to involve them in the choice of specific topics or tasks to be undertaken.

Clearly define the problem or topic to be addressed and the nature of the task confronting the group. Tell them the objectives or enlist their aid in defining or modifying the objectives.

ENCOURAGING GROUP PARTICIPATION

Arrange seating in such a way that group members can freely talk to each other.

Try to ensure that group members are prepared for the discussion by notifying them of the topic in advance, prescribing prior activities or pre-reading assignments.

Resist the temptation to talk too much and provide all the answers. Given enough time to become comfortable and to think, most group members find that they can contribute usefully to each other's knowledge and skills.

Be aware of the stages that groups pass through and be prepared to help the group through difficult phases. Use gently probing questions that focus the discussion and encourage quieter group members to speak.

Be aware of the various roles that members of the group are assuming, and of the ways in which they participate, and be prepared to help them to learn effective ways to contribute to the discussion or task.

FINISHING OFF THE DISCUSSION

Warn students 10 minutes before the end of time so that they can come to some conclusions or closure in their discussion or task.

Summarize, or encourage the students to summarize, the discussion and highlight the main points discussed and the main achievements in relation to the objectives.

Review the work that still needs to be done and set the task for the next meeting.

Specific strategies for encouraging group discussion are many. One of the most relevant and effective strategies in use in nurse education is role play (e.g. Reed and Procter, 1993).

ROLE PLAY

Role play is a teaching strategy in which students take the roles of participants in a situation. The general aim is to enable students to experience situations and learn to deal with them before they meet them in real life.

PURPOSES OF ROLE PLAY

ACTIVITY

You may have used role play or considered using it in your teaching. Make a list of the purposes or learning objectives which role play can help nursing students achieve.

FEEDBACK

The main purpose of role play is to enable students to practise skills or to experience their own and others' reactions to particular situations they will face in nursing practice. Undoubtedly, these same skills and reactions can be encountered in real-life situations, such as ward or community work; however, nursing practice deals with sensitive issues and situations which may involve risk to patients. Opportunities to practise in simulated or lifelike situations are needed before students can apply their skills in caring for real patients or solving real problems. Specific purposes for which role play is often used include:

- learning communication skills, e.g. interviewing a patient or relatives;
- learning procedural skills, e.g. taking blood pressure or assisting in the operating theatre;
- learning about relationships between people, e.g. the members of the health team, and the factors that assist or impede their ability to work together;
- exploring emotions involved in certain types of situation or with certain types of behaviour, e.g. caring for terminally ill patients, sick children and their families;
- trying out new behaviour, skills or attitudes in situations which resemble reality but which allow for feedback and entail no risks to the patient or the student;
- enabling students to reflect on practice.

An important aspect of the role play is that even though players are acting a role they should be free to express their own reactions and feelings spontaneously within that role. Players do not rehearse parts or learn scripts but make up their own responses within the general scenario, as the role play goes on. People vary in their ability to put themselves into a role but, with support, encouragement and an informal relaxed atmosphere generated in a group who are used to working together, most students find that they can participate to some extent. Some roles generate significant reactions within some players and some groups, so a vital component of all role play should be the 'de-roling' which follows. In this de-roling, players are given an opportunity to discuss their feelings and reactions to the role and to differentiate between their real feelings and those that were only a part of the role. It is the teacher's responsibility to ensure that the discussion following the role play contributes to the students' achievement of the learning objectives, and provides an opportunity for resolution or follow-up of any problems that may have surfaced in the individual or the group.

PLANNING AND CONDUCTING A ROLE PLAY

Successful role plays don't just happen, they have to be planned. The degree of guidance given to players and the group will depend to a large extent on the objectives of the session and on the level of experience of the group. However, the basic steps to be followed in planning a role play remain fairly constant.

1. Set objectives for the role play

Prepare the students by telling them what the role play is supposed to achieve in general terms. Make sure that the students have enough background knowledge and that they can relate the role play to familiar experiences.

Example of objectives for a role play

- To develop skills in providing medication instructions to patients on discharge from hospital.
- To identify the difficulties inherent in transferring an elderly patient from the hospital environment to self-care when several medications are necessary.

- To explore the responsibilities of the patient, the doctor, the nurse and the family in ensuring optimal care.
- To experience the feelings of an elderly patient who is being discharged from hospital on a new treatment regimen.

2. Prepare a scenario

The scenario is a brief outline of the situation that provides the setting, the problem or situation involved and the motives of the players. Each player is told something of his or her own motives but not of the motives of the other players (as is usually the case in real-life situations). You must provide enough detail to get the players started but not so much that the players have no room to express their own emotions and reactions in the roles.

Example of a scenario

- Setting:
  By the bedside. An 83-year-old man is being discharged from hospital after 3 weeks as an inpatient undergoing treatment for digitalis intoxication, cardiac arrhythmia and congestive cardiac failure. His dosage of digitalis has been halved and he is taking a stronger diuretic and some potassium supplements, and vitamin supplements at various times of the day. He understands from hearing medical students talk about his case that he was ill because he had been taking too high a dose of his heart tablets before coming into hospital. He lives in a self-contained flat behind his daughter's house but is alone most of the day because his daughter's family go to work and school.
- Players:
  The old man: You are slightly deaf. You are afraid that your daughter's family don't want you back because you are a burden to them. You do not understand why you have to take all these new tablets, especially since you understand that your recent illness was caused by too much of one of them. You don't like to ask the doctors too many questions because they always seem to be busy so you have asked the nurse to explain what tablets should be taken and when you can stop taking them.
  The nurse: You are a junior nurse and you are surprised that the patient is asking about his medication. You assumed that it was the doctor's responsibility to explain this to the patient; in any case you have not been very involved with this patient's management and

are not sure of the reasons for his change of medication. You decide to talk to the patient's daughter when she comes to collect him because the old man is a little deaf and you don't have too much time to spend explaining. The doctor is in the clinic and unable to come to the ward. The head nurse has to provide a report on your work and you are reluctant to reveal that you do not know how to handle the situation.

The daughter: You are worried because your father almost died before he came into hospital and you are afraid that he will become ill at home again and that you won't be able to look after him. You haven't seen his doctor in the hospital because he is usually not around at visiting hours but you seek reassurance from the nurse who seems to be looking after your father.

The head nurse: You are aware of the situation and have decided to see how the nurse handles the situation before stepping in to help her out. You intend to discuss the problem with her later and point out how she could improve her skills in this area.

3. Assign roles

Players should volunteer to take part. Other group members should act as observers to take note of interesting events in the role play for discussion afterward. While players are taking a few minutes to prepare for their roles, observers could be discussing the issues or points that should be looked out for in that scenario with those particular objectives. Alternatively, you can provide the observers with a list of things to watch for – this list will depend on the objectives of the session.

4. Carry out the role play

Players should respond spontaneously to each other for as long as the activity is important and relevant. Take care to stop the role play before it becomes boring or before so much happens that you won't be able to discuss it all. Of course you should be sensitive to what is happening in the role play and only stop it when it gets to a natural break in the interactions.

If you have videotape equipment it is very helpful to record the role play so that it can be referred to during the following discussion.

5. Follow-up discussion

The purpose of this discussion is to allow students to talk about, understand and receive feedback on the experience they have just had.

Players should try to describe their view of what happened and the reactions engendered in themselves and other players. These views should then be compared with information gathered by the observers. Discussion should try to identify the patterns in relationships and the causes and effects of the events in the role play and then transfer these patterns to relevant real-life experiences. The role play should always be tied back into the real situation in which students will eventually find themselves.

ROLE REVERSAL

This is an alternative technique (Brookfield, 1991) that you could try when you decide that students would benefit by observing another person in the role play who is playing the role the student normally plays. It is a powerful technique and is often used in cross-cultural education or negotiation seminars in administration.

ACTIVITY

Identify a situation in your teaching area which might be effectively illustrated by a role play.

Write a scenario for the role play and try it out with your students.

FEEDBACK

Use the checklist in Figure 4.1 to assess how effective your role play was.

If your answer to any of these questions was 'no' then you should reread the section on role play and check each part of your role-play exercise to see where you could improve it. Feedback from students or colleagues who participated in the role play should help you here.

Don't give up if you have one unsuccessful experience – role play is a method that improves with practice by both teacher and students.

REFLECTIVE ACTIVITIES

CRITICAL INCIDENT

The critical incident is described in Chapter 8 as an assessment method, and this is its most familiar use. In this chapter, we recognize that the critical incident technique is a teaching as well as a testing method. Smith and Russell (1993) provide arguments for its use as a developmental method in undergraduate education to bring to life the linkages between theory and practice. They note its value in strengthening student–teacher relationships and the close similarity of the method with Benner's (1984, p 299–300) work with exemplars.

Brookfield (1991, p 31) defines critical incidents as 'brief written reports compiled by students about their experience of learning'. He has been able to demonstrate to teachers by the use of a critical incident questionnaire how they can 'tune in' to how their students are learning. The questions he uses are framed so that students give descriptions of specific events. This has the advantage of being non-threatening to students and closer to their real experiences than a series of abstract questions on the nature of teaching.

	Yes	No
Were the objectives clear to participants at the beginning?	☐	☐
Was the scenario good enough to promote the behaviour you wanted to demonstrate?	☐	☐
Were the players able to play their roles?	☐	☐
Were the players able to describe their experiences and attitudes to the group?	☐	☐
Did students gain appropriate feedback on their skills or attitudes?	☐	☐
Did the observers observe relevant information and report it to the group?	☐	☐
Was the group able to draw some conclusions about the causes and effects of the behaviours demonstrated in the role play?	☐	☐
Were the objectives of the role play achieved?	☐	☐
Did the group enjoy the experience and find it worthwhile?	☐	☐

Figure 4.1 Checklist for assessing the effectiveness of a role play.

ACTIVITY

Why not try Brookfield's method yourself before you use it in one of your classes. Nurse educators seldom have time to stop and reflect on what they are learning about their teaching. While you are answering the critical incident questionnaire, make a few notes on your reactions to the questions. Could you adapt this set of questions for your students?

Directions

Think back over a recent teaching session you had with your students. Describe, in as specific, concrete and honest a fashion as you can, the following details of this experience:

- the incident (or incidents) that you recall as being most exciting and rewarding – a teaching 'high' for you – a time when you felt that something important and significant was happening to you as a teacher;
- the incident (or incidents) that you recall as being the most distressing or disappointing for you – a teaching 'low' – a time when you felt despair or frustration about your teaching skills;
- the characteristics and behaviours of students that you found most helpful in your teaching – give specific examples of events in which these were observable;
- the characteristics and behaviours of student that you found hindered your teaching – give specific examples of events in which these were observable;
- those times when you felt valued and affirmed as a teacher and why this was so;
- those times when you felt demeaned and patronized as a teacher and why this was so;
- the most important insights you had about the nature of effective learning;
- the most important insights you had about yourself as a teacher;
- what pleased you most in the teaching you experienced;
- what were the most painful aspects in the teaching you experienced.

(Source: adapted from Brookfield, 1991, p 32)

FEEDBACK

You could debrief your responses to another teacher to obtain maximum personal benefit from the exercise. You could also compare your responses with those of your students. By changing 'teaching' to 'learning' in the questions you could give the questionnaire to your class and follow it with a review of the responses to the 10 questions by asking students to identify any common themes. For example, which are the most and the least helpful learning experiences and what advice would you give to a teacher about which methods seem the most helpful to students?

Helping your students to reflect on their learning can put them in touch with ways to take control of their continuing learning as professionals. If they are willing to admit that there is pain and anxiety as well as pleasure in learning they are better prepared to face the learning of new and different roles as science and technology bring increasing information and professional challenges and responsibilities.

Critical incidents have a wider use than the one we have just pursued. Smith and Russell (1993) have used the technique for a number of purposes. Using critical reflection they applaud the value of the critical incident method in 'entering the student's world' by discovering and using incidents that students themselves identify as critical. The précis below has been drawn from their full description of their method (Smith and Russell, 1993). Reading the whole chapter provides insights into innovative and sensitive teaching and learning.

The particular adaptation of the method required students to record a particularly memorable incident. They were also asked to note the associated feelings or thoughts they recalled. These anonymous accounts were then collected by the staff prior to a workshop where several selected incidents judged to offer valuable learning would form the focus. Themes from the incidents were identified by the staff. Specially chosen content and learning strategies focused on the incidents and themes were followed by debate and questioning by the students. An interesting strategy is used to look at what the authors call 'snapshots' of experience, to prompt the students to question the relation of theory and practice through a series of questions.

- What happened in this incident?
- How can it be explained?
- Are there any other conceptual frameworks which might increase our understanding?

The interweaving of reflection on experience and analysis of actual incidents critical to students provides a unique adaptation to the critical incident method.

JOURNALLING

Private records of how students make sense and feel about their practice and their learning have become popular as the autonomy of learners has become valued and respected. Journalling provides an example of students seeing learning from their perspective rather than from the teacher's. Ludinsky (1990) calls the process of journal writing, 'reflective withdrawal'. Modra (1989) describes learning journals which encourage critical thinking in distance education. MacDonald's (1993) purpose was to explore the concept of caring and his personal journey in uncovering his feelings and beliefs about his caring practice. After becoming immersed in the literature on caring and finding an array of words describing 'attributes of compassion and emotional involvement', MacDonald puzzled over questions such as the following:

- Do caregivers invariably utilize and practise them?
- Should nurses be expected to bring all of these caring traits into clinical caring all of the time?
- Are these theorists discussing realities that carers can relate to, or are they discussing altruistic 'academic' caring that is at odds with clinical practice?

MacDonald describes how journalling proved helpful in reflecting on his recorded observations and personal notes while also linking these with the literature. He is able to speak to his journal and unravel his confusion in a scrupulously honest account, battling with feelings of 'non-caring' as well as caring. His conclusions show that critical reflection and an emancipatory approach are possible through journalling and can be a valuable process used by professionals as well as students.

As a registered nurse, MacDonald chose his own way of journalling. For your students you would need to provide guidance in explaining the difference between diaries and journals. Most students would be familiar with diaries, the personal recording of what happens each day and how they feel about themselves, other people and the events. Although there are a variety of ways of journalling, a theme, a critical question or a learning need is usually the focus and the progressive experiences are examined in the light of the focus.

STORYTELLING

As most nurses know, experienced nurses have accumulated a vast amount of information from their day-to-day practice activities and observations. Students, as well, are building and storing information from their experiences of practice but also from their academic studies. What sense do they make from the melding of the two sources together? What help do they get to unravel the tangled impressions they might have? What opportunities do they have to express their inexperience in a supportive, reflective and non-threatening group?

Storytelling as a learning strategy might appear to be a contradiction in terms. Nurses have never been slow in telling their stories and, at the informal level, storytelling has been a feature of the private and personal nursing world. Lindesmith and McWeeny (1994) have found that storytelling can be a powerful learning strategy when it is understood as a reflective practice shared by a small group of committed listeners.

Lindesmith and McWeeny begin the strategy by the facilitator first telling a story as a demonstration of the process. This has the effect of encouraging, 'giving permission' and showing acceptance of stories and storytellers.

The guidelines for facilitators include the following.

- Create an environment conducive to storytelling.
- Model the experience through your own story.
- Invite the sharing of stories around a programme theme.
- Encourage attentive listening to each other's stories.
- Initiate group discussion about the experience.

Students may feel that the story they tell has to be about something remarkable or especially noteworthy for one reason or another. They may devalue the experience and information that is derived from practice and therefore dismiss any stories which are not 'important'. Storytelling is a splendid opportunity for students to realize that there is a richness of experience, knowledge and skill embedded and sometimes hidden in practice. The skill of making that manifest through reflection is one of the most important teaching skills.

INDEPENDENT LEARNING

Independent learning is a term that creates a lot of confusion. Perhaps the easiest way to define it is as a process in which learners are encouraged to take increasing personal responsibility for achieving learning objectives through their own efforts and at their own pace.

Some examples of independent learning are:

- self-instructional learning units;
- continuing education through reading or other resource-based activities;
- elective subjects within training courses;
- correspondence courses.

The independence of the learner varies according to who makes the decisions about what to learn and how to learn it.

Total independence of the learner occurs when the learner decides on the objectives of the learning, the methods for learning and the criteria for assessment – in other words, when learning is self-directed. Total dependence of the learner occurs when the teacher decides on the objectives, methods and criteria for assessment – in other words, when learning is teacher-directed.

A continuum of learning which ranges from totally student-directed to totally teacher-directed can be described as in Table 4.1.

Table 4.1 Continuum of independent learning

Student-directed learning	Student decides objectives, methods and assessment.
	Student decides objectives and methods. Teacher decides assessment in consultation with student.
	Student and teacher discuss and negotiate on objectives, methods and assessment.
Increasing independence	Teacher decides objectives. Student chooses methods. Teacher decides criteria for assessment.
	Teacher decides objectives and assessment and recommends a variety of methods.
Teacher-directed learning	Teacher decides objectives, methods and assessments.

Very few professional training courses are totally self-directed. However, there are advantages in encouraging students to be more self-directed in their learning.

- If learners set themselves problems to solve or tasks to perform they are more motivated by curiosity or interest to learn the relevant information and to remember it. Teachers can contribute by providing guidance on the scope of problems which can realistically be tackled within specific time periods.
- Self-directed learners learn how to learn as well as just learning facts. New facts continually replace the old facts learned in training and nurses may quickly become out of date unless they know how to discover and learn new facts as they become available. Continuing education depends heavily on the nurse's ability to recognize what she/he needs to learn and to seek opportunities for learning it formally or informally.

- Self-directed learners become more experienced in working without close supervision so that when they enter their jobs as nurses they are more confident of their own abilities and do not have to rely on someone else to tell them what to do. If they have had experience in self-assessment and self-determination of what they need to know they will recognize their own limitations and know how to overcome them.
- Self-directed learners come to realize that the classroom or training school is not the only place where learning occurs. Many important sources of knowledge and skills learning exist in everyday activities in the home and community. Self-directed learners are encouraged to use these resources instead of relying on information provided only by the teachers. Knowing how to use these resources will be an important part of the nurse's job.

Learning in nursing schools is largely teacher-directed, whereas most learning that nurses experience after they have finished training must be self-directed. Nursing training should prepare students to be self-directed so that they can take responsibility for their own continuing education when they are working in the community or hospital.

ACTIVITY

Write down as many ways as you can think of to help your students to become self-directed or independent learners.

FEEDBACK

Introducing the idea of independent learning to students is not always easy. Some may have experienced a degree of self-directed learning in their previous secondary or tertiary education and may be familiar with it and able to benefit from it from the beginning. Many students, however, are not confident enough to take responsibility for their own learning. They expect the teacher to tell them what to learn, how to learn it and whether they have learned it well. It may be wise to introduce independent learning experiences gradually. This allows both you and your students to become familiar with the particular demands and responsibilities of the new roles that you are required to play. Coombs and her co-workers (1981) have described a workshop that gradually introduces nurses to concepts of self-directed learning. Some other specific approaches that you might like to try are listed below.

Offer students a choice of topic

Of course there are some things in nursing that students must all know or be able to do and you must help students to master those 'must know' objectives. However, there are also many topics which are enriching, which contribute to the nurse's ability to do the job but which are not essential for it. No student will ever be able to learn all there is to know about nursing and so, once the essential knowledge and skills have been mastered, students can be offered a choice of topics which particularly interest them. Most schools offer elective terms or programmes in their curricula, but electives can also be offered within specific subjects. For example, students might undertake a special reading assignment relevant to a patient for whom they have been given responsibility, or they may be given the opportunity to participate in and report on a community aid project.

Your student would, of course, need to discuss the aims, scope, resources and criteria for assessment of the independent project with you before starting, but within certain guidelines could be encouraged to develop the study as independently as possible.

Vary the scope and depth of topics to be covered

Basic material can be taught in class and more advanced material can be provided in libraries or resource centres to allow students to follow up material in which they have a greater interest. Students could be encouraged to go beyond class work and to further their skills or knowledge by spending free time engaged in extra reading or activities with you or a group of other interested students. Incentives for this extra work could take the form of opportunity to earn extra credits towards the course assessment. Swanson and Dalsing (1980) have described the use of independent study in this way as a curriculum expander.

Provide alternative methods for learning

Providing a variety of resources and experiences for learning helps students to discover which methods they prefer and which types of activity or resources help them to learn best. For example, some students learn best by reading, some by listening or discussing. If students are given the opportunity to try a variety of methods they will learn more about how to learn effectively in the future.

Provide students with problems to solve

Students who are involved actively in learning through solving problems will remember what they have learned better than they would if the same information had been given to them by the teacher. In addition, they will have learned an approach to solving problems which will be very useful to them when they are presented with nursing problems in the course of their work.

As students become more adept at the process of problem-solving they may discover or generate problems for themselves to solve as part of their elective or practicum studies. Problem-solving is an important approach to the development of independent learners because it requires students to proceed through the following steps, seeking answers to their own questions as they go.

- What is the problem – what are the components of the problem?
- What information or skills will be needed to solve the problem?
- Where can the information be found?
- How can the necessary skills be developed?
- How should the knowledge and skills be applied to solve the problem?
- Did the solution work – might there have been a better one?

Since the problem-solving process depends on students identifying, finding and applying needed information and skills, the teacher should act only as guide and adviser rather than as giver of information or provider of solutions.

Consider using self-instructional course units

If self-instructional programmes are available they allow students to learn at their own pace and at the time of their choosing whether a teacher is present or not. Students can use these materials to learn basic information so that the time they spend with the teacher can be used to help them overcome special difficulties or to increase their level of skill or understanding. The student becomes more independent because it is her/his responsibility to discuss individual learning needs with the teacher rather than relying on the teacher to prescribe everything that should be learned.

Provide opportunities for self-assessment

Students should have frequent opportunities to assess their own performance. The ability to set criteria for personal performance and to gauge performance against those criteria is a critical professional skill for the nurse. Initially students may need guidance in setting criteria and in evaluating themselves against those criteria, but if results of self-assessment are checked with the teacher and guidance is provided students can learn to improve the accuracy of self-assessments. A useful adjunct to self-directed learning and self-assessment is the contracting system, in which the student contracts with the instructor to achieve specific objectives. The objectives and methods for the study are agreed in consultation and the student is encouraged to develop criteria by which his or her achievement of objectives of the study can be judged. Once the criteria have been agreed to by both parties then the student is able to assess his or her own work accurately. This system also allows students to contract for certain grades. Kruse and Fagerbarger (1982) have described the application of contracting in nursing education.

Get to know your students

If you know your students as individuals and if you demonstrate interest and concern for their needs and their professional development, students will feel more able to take risks, to reveal their uncertainties and their difficulties, in the confidence that you are there to help rather than to judge. Development of self-confidence in learning that leads to the ability to be a self-directed professional depends on the students' preparedness to take these risks. This is particularly true in the area of clinical learning, which is a source of anxiety for most students and many teachers.

ACTIVITY

You will have recognized by now that the teacher's tasks in self-directed or independent learning are quite different from the teacher's tasks in traditional teacher-directed learning.

Complete Table 4.2(a), which contrasts the two sets of tasks in each of the areas of educational planning.

Table 4.2(a)   Contrast of learning tasks

	Teacher's tasks in teacher-directed learning	Teacher's tasks in student-related learning
Objectives		
Content		
Methods		
Feedback		
Assessment		

FEEDBACK

Check your answers with Table 4.2(b).

Table 4.2(b)   Contrast of learning tasks

	Teacher's tasks in teacher-directed learning	Teacher's tasks in student-directed learning
Objectives	Define learning objectives	Help students to define appropriate learning objectives or problems to investigate
Content	Provide information in lectures, handouts, books	Act as a resource to guide students seeking information which will help them achieve their objectives
Methods	Design teaching methods and resources to help students learn	Make resources available and act as a guide to available facilities which students might seek
Feedback	Provide feedback on performance	Encourage students to provide their own feedback before submitting work to the teacher for assessment
Assessment	Assess student's achievements of learning objectives	Work with students to achieve a mutual assessment of the strengths and weaknesses of their independent study project

The teacher's role in student-directed learning is mainly as a guide, a helper and a source of encouragement to strengthen the students' own efforts and abilities. As students become more independent they will have less need for guidance, help and encouragement and will be able to find their own way to suitable resources and provide quite accurate judgements of the quality of their own work. That is the ultimate goal of independent learning.

If all this is beginning to worry you because it seems too different from your usual practice or because you doubt your students' ability, be encouraged by the following three points.

- Independent learning should not be isolated learning. Students will always need opportunities to interact with their teachers and with each other. Learning how to participate in a group and how to give and receive support and feedback are essential for the development of independent learning skills.
- Independent learning is an important skill for nurses to develop but it is only one of many skills they must have. You should provide some opportunities for students to develop it but you need not do all your teaching that way. A variety of teaching and learning methods is essential. Too much independent learning can be just as frustrating or boring as too many lectures.

- Independent learning does not require something extra or special from your students. What it requires is that they learn to use experience and skills that they already possess.

When students attend a nursing school they know they have much to learn and they feel that the teachers have all the answers to their questions. They tend to disregard their own knowledge as irrelevant or unimportant in comparison with that of the teacher. You as the teacher must try to help them recognize the importance of what they can contribute to their own and other students' learning.

USING MODERN EDUCATIONAL MEDIA

The first edition of this book contained a chapter on using learning resources, including educational media. Since that chapter was written, there has been an educational technology revolution which promises to change dramatically the processes of education itself. A single chapter in a book such as this can no longer do justice to the possibilities confronting the teacher.

Computers have entered the classroom, the health-care system, the home and the office to an extent not dreamed of 10 years ago.

Most students leaving modern schools can be assumed to be computer-literate; many universities are introducing computer-literacy as a prerequisite for graduation. Academic staff are increasingly retraining to be able to exploit computer technology in their research, in the classroom and on the international information superhighway. For information on the latest in these areas, your best resource will be your own institution's library, your information technology service and your educational media services.

Helpful overviews are also provided in Tinkler *et al.*, 1994; Laurillard, 1993; Hannafin and Peck, 1988; and Latchem, Williamson and Henderson-Lancett, 1993.

SUMMARY

This chapter has covered a variety of teaching and learning methods each of which is suited to different educational needs. Of course there is some overlap between methods and what they can achieve. You should aim to use a variety of methods to give your students practice in working in a variety of ways, and you should, if your facilities permit, use those methods best suited to your learning objectives and to your personal talents and preferences.

To summarize the main points we have covered in this unit, try the next activity.

ACTIVITY

Make a list of the main educational purposes for using each of the following teaching/learning methods.

- Lectures
- Small-group tutorials
- Role play
- Critical incidents
- Journalling
- Storytelling
- Independent learning.

FEEDBACK

Each of these methods has special capabilities that make it more useful for some types of learning than others. You, the teacher, must choose which methods you prefer to use in your class. While some methods may be best suited to some objectives they may be unsuitable for other reasons unique to your situation. For this reason it is not possible to lay down absolute rules that will help you to decide. The following should be used only as a guide.

Use lectures if you want to:

- provide a structure to guide students in learning a topic;
- give an overview of a complex topic;
- provide perspective and emphasize parts of the topic;
- provide information which is not available elsewhere.

Supplement the lecture with handouts, discussions and audiovisual aids when appropriate.

Use small-group tutorials if you want to:

- involve students as active participants;
- develop skills in teamwork and co-operation;
- develop manual or communication skills;
- provide practice in applying knowledge to problems or tasks;
- promote new ideas and attitudes;
- allow for clarifying understanding of a topic.

Use role-play activities if you want to:

- explore emotions involved with a topic;
- try new behaviour and attitudes in a safe setting similar to the real one;
- explore relationships and why people behave as they do.

Use critical incidents if you want to:

- explore an aspect of learning or practice;
- involve students in reflection;
- help students analyse theories, feelings, beliefs and values;
- help students come to terms with the ambiguities in practice;
- encourage critical thinking.

Use journalling and storytelling if you want to:

- encourage exploration of theoretical concepts and own practice;
- help students practise 'reflective withdrawal';
- encourage critical thinking.

Use modern educational media in the most appropriate ways to support the learning objectives of the programme. Modern media can make a valuable contribution to all teaching methods if they are well designed and their use is planned as an integral component of the learning experience.

Use independent learning if you want to:

- help students learn how to rely on their own judgement;
- help students become increasingly independent;
- encourage students to learn outside the classroom;
- prepare students for lifelong continuing education.

Fostering clinical learning

5

INTRODUCTION

In the previous chapter we included the teaching methods you could use when helping students to learn. Discussion in small groups, role plays, critical incidents and some of the other methods are also appropriate for fostering clinical learning. In this chapter we will add to those methods and include ways to plan and organize clinical learning sessions. As you go through this chapter you might find it helpful to refer to the assessment of clinical performance in Chapter 8.

When you have finished this chapter you should be able to foster clinical learning through:

- preparing students for clinical learning – briefing or pre-conference;
- reinforcing learning during practice – reflection-in-practice;
- reflecting on practice – debriefing or post-conference.

In the 10 years since the first edition of this book there have been many changes in the way nurse teachers plan, organize, conduct and evaluate clinical learning. As nursing education systems in many countries have become part of the tertiary education structures of universities and colleges an intense spotlight has been thrown on clinical education. What the public and professional glare has shown is that, regardless of the undoubted value of the increase in the theoretical programme, the benefits of learning in real situations are now recognized for their educational as well as their practical significance.

Coming to terms with what is involved in clinical learning has assumed increasing significance as programmes consider the implications of costs, teaching resources and the organization of clinical programmes. Role clarification has become essential to identify the roles of, for example, nurse teachers with a clinical teaching load, preceptors, mentors, lecturer-practitioners, nurse teachers with clinical liaison responsibilities, clinical staff with teaching interests and clinical assessors.

Compared with the challenges presented by the complexities of clinical learning and teaching, the relatively stable environment of the classroom has never been so inviting!

However, the classroom is not out of bounds or excluded from helping students to find meaning in what they are doing and thinking in clinical practice. Showing students how to link their clinical work with what they are learning in the classroom and recognizing the practical knowledge students have derived from practice are teaching skills that know no boundaries of location. The criteria of relevance, the learner and the perspective on nursing that we identified as important in selecting content (Chapter 2) applies throughout the programme. Applying theory to practice with those criteria in mind has become an important and necessary day-to-day skill of every nurse teacher.

DEFINITION OF CLINICAL LEARNING

There are a number of definitions of clinical learning that include one or several facets of the subject such as transfer of knowledge to practical situations, all the directed activities of the student in clinical practice and the socialization of nurses into the culture of nursing. The definitions tend to reflect the particular theoretical or ideological standpoint of the authors who give them. While there is no argument with this, for this chapter we have tended to remain with the definition (and its rationale) that we included in the first edition of this text.

A broad definition of clinical learning is **learning that occurs in settings similar to the ones in which the student will eventually work.**

Adopting this broader definition allows us to shift the focus from purely bedside activities (the traditional meaning of the word 'clinical') to the broader range of activities in which nurses will find themselves involved. These other activities include community services of various kinds and the variety of contexts in which nursing is practised.

Different countries or even different institutions within countries have evolved different systems for providing clinical education. The differences lie in the extent to which the system of nurse education functions freely within an autonomous school of nursing or is less able to direct its own activities. One problem that most systems seem to have in common is the difficulty of helping students make the transition from classroom to clinic or ward and from knowledge acquisition to application of that knowledge in the solution of clinical problems, the 'theory–practice divide'. Problems may be further compounded by conflicts that arise between the student nurse's educational and service roles and the expectations of clinical educators and supervisors in relation to those roles. Good communication between school-based nurse educators, clinical supervisors and students is a vital component of clinical learning and should be foremost in mind when the objectives and methods of clinical learning are being considered.

AIMS OF CLINICAL EDUCATION

ACTIVITY

Clinical education is vital for the preparation of professional nurses who can function competently and independently in a diversity of nursing situations. Make a list of the main aims of clinical education.

FEEDBACK

Much has been written about the aims of clinical education (for example, see Carpenito and Duespohl, 1985; Infante, 1985; Watts, 1990; White and Ewan, 1991; Reilly and Oermann, 1992. The general aims for clinical education seem to fall into five main areas:

- to help students to learn skills they will need as nurses to practice intelligently and reflectively in a changing health-care system and to gain an understanding of the principles underlying those skills (Fawcett and McQueen, 1994);
- to help students learn to deal with situations and people they will meet in the nursing role and to understand the wider context in which their practice takes place (Perry, 1991);
- to provide students with supervised practice in applying their factual knowledge and learned skills to the solution of real problems in the practical situation of health care (Infante, 1985);
- to help students to understand the nature of clinical practice and to gain confidence in their own abilities to carry out their role; to guide the student in the transition from student to independent professional (Packer, 1994);
- to enable students to work with senior practitioners who can model appropriate behaviour and attitudes, and to expose students to experiences which will help to shape their attitudes in desirable directions (Wiseman, 1994).

These are some of the purposes for which clinical education can be used and your own experience in a clinical education programme could, no doubt, add other purposes which are specific to your students, the programme and its conceptual framework. However, unless the clinical experience is planned with these explicit aims in mind it can be a frustrating experience that does not achieve its full potential.

SOME PROBLEMS OF CLINICAL EDUCATION

ACTIVITY

Think of the clinical education that you have experienced, either as a student or teacher. From your own experience, identify the problems which can arise in clinical learning and therefore the characteristics of effective clinical experiences that avoid those problems.

FEEDBACK

From your experience as a teacher, the problems you most commonly identified could be shared by many of your colleagues. Examples might be as follows.

- The clinical learning environment is unpredictable and uncertain with rapid changes so that there can be little control over the clinical learning experiences for students.
- Planning for clinical teaching requires a knowledge of the patients or clients in the students' clinical assignments and knowledge of the students' level of learning and experience.
- The nurse teacher is a guest in the clinical area and clinical experiences are sometimes difficult to arrange because the clinical setting is also a service setting and full-time staff are usually concerned with their patient-care responsibilities; role conflict can sometimes be an impediment to negotiations for student placements.
- Your role as a teacher in the clinical setting may expand to be a manager, assessor, an advocate, a facilitator and a guide for students in unfamiliar environments of ward, clinical or community facilities.

- The time you spend in commuting from one health agency to another to supervise students in different locations may be out of proportion to the time you actually spend teaching or supervising.
- You may feel that the expectation for you to be clinically credible across a wide spectrum of clinical care where your students practise is unrealistic.

The list could continue and, in addition, your students have probably made you aware, from time to time, of their problems with clinical learning. These might include the following.

- Clinical supervisors may not be fully aware of the objectives of the placement or of the background knowledge and skills that your students have when they arrive; in situations in which students are needed to fulfil service roles they may even be assigned to clinical areas in which they have had no background learning; students often have little opportunity to achieve the objectives for which the placement was intended.
- Students themselves may be unprepared for or ignorant of the objectives or specific purposes of the placement and therefore unable to properly direct their own learning efforts; they may be uncomfortable in the clinical setting and have uncertainties about their roles and others' expectations of them.
- Students are sometimes critical of clinical teachers, who may misuse the unique learning opportunities provided through clinical education by teaching students in the same way as they would in the classroom. Handovers at report time may become mini-lectures, instead of an opportunity for the students to practise giving a report and getting feedback about the care given to patients assigned to them.
- Students can sometimes be the proverbial 'meat in the sandwich' and may miss many valuable opportunities for guidance and feedback because, in some organizational frameworks for clinical teaching, the respective roles of school-based nurse educators and service-based clinical supervisors give rise to uncertainties over role definition and acceptance of responsibility for various aspects of training.
- Students at times feel that their assessors do not realize how much they have actually learned nor how they are using reasoning and problem-solving skills because the assessment system tests only what can be observed and measured objectively.

- Students can be fearful of the dual roles of clinical teachers as both teachers and assessors, and are unsure of the dividing line between their clinical learning and their clinical assessment.
- There are many distractions in the clinical situation: the complexities of the caring environment, the presence of a patient in pain or distress and the competing responsibilities of caring and learning can be confusing and deeply troubling for both students and teachers.

How can these problems and others which you may have identified be overcome?

In brief, most clinical education in the health professions falls into three broad phases:

1. **preparation for practice**: skill learning and practice and pre-conference or briefing;
2. **practice with supervision**: 'reflection-in-practice';
3. **post-practice discussion**: post-conference or debriefing 'reflection on practice'

PREPARATION FOR PRACTICE

LEARNING THE SKILLS OF PRACTICE

This includes:

- demonstration and practice of skills or techniques in a skills laboratory;
- providing simulated experiences;
- briefing or pre-conference.

Demonstration and practice of skills and techniques

Frequently, as part of the preparation for practice, the teacher will be called upon to demonstrate skills or techniques. Inexperienced teachers sometimes fall into the trap of assuming that demonstration is sufficient to ensure that students know how to proceed with practising the skill. This is not necessarily so. There are three steps in a successful demonstration: demonstration, followed by supervised practice of the components of the task, followed by return demonstration in which the students demonstrate that they are able to integrate the components into performance of the task.

It is worth taking a little time out here to look at the characteristics of an effective demonstration. The following checklist may be useful if you have to plan demonstrations from time to time.

- **What are the purposes or objectives of your demonstration?** If your objectives require students to be able to perform the task you are demonstrating then you must also provide opportunities for practise and feedback.
- **What can you do to increase the students' involvement in the demonstration?** Almost by definition a demonstration causes the audience to be passive. Learners learn better when they are actively involved. You should therefore plan your demonstration so that students are required to become involved in it in some way rather than to just watch. Ask some students to help, some to act as observers, provide written handouts and questions to guide students' thinking and observations, stop the demonstration at suitable points for questions and discussion and make sure that every student has a good view of what is happening.
- **What are the main points you want to make in the demonstration?** Begin the demonstration by telling students briefly what you are about to do and summarizing the main points they should watch for. You could choose some of the students to note down their observations at those key points and you should also point these out as they occur. By providing such a 'road map' through the demonstration you can ensure that students do not get lost in the technical details, which might be likely to distract their attention.
  At the end of the demonstration ask the students to summarize the lessons learned.
- **What resources will you require to carry out the demonstration?** Obviously you will assemble and check all the necessary technical equipment or materials for your demonstration beforehand. It is also worth thinking about whether any additional resources, such as diagrams or handouts, will help the students to get the most benefit from the demonstration. For example, you could provide an observation checklist that requires the students to fill in their observations against certain questions or headings on the sheet.
- **Is the relevance of the demonstration clear?** Since demonstrations can be quite complex and time-consuming you should be sure that the demonstration is actually necessary for the achievement of your objectives. You should also make sure that students understand the relevance of the demonstration to what they are learning to do. Otherwise they may find it confusing or boring.

- **Have you provided opportunities for supervised practice and return demonstration?** Once you are satisfied with the students' level of skill and understanding of the basic principles applied to clinical practice then the students can be moved on through the next level of clinical education, which is practice under supervision in a real setting, most often the ward or community centre.

Providing simulated experiences

A simulation is a useful alternative to an experience in the real world for students who need to gain confidence and skills before giving care to patients and clients. The simulation needs to be conducted in the safety of a controlled setting, usually with a simulated client and a representation of the client's environment.

ACTIVITY

You are planning to involve your students in a simulated exercise to give them practice in explaining and negotiating with a patient about to be discharged on the advisability of after-care and home visits. How will you plan for and conduct the simulation?

FEEDBACK

Structuring the simulated exercise

First, you will need to collect information about the client and the problem, the medical condition, the nursing problem, the home and surrounding environment. This could be material from slides, overheads, notes and written reports.

Next, the students need to be prepared, particularly if they have not been involved in a simulated exercise before. You could explain that they will all take turns in interviewing the client, and that they can opt for 'time out' if they get stuck and need to review how they are going. Some students could exhibit frustration as they find their skills are not up to standard, and could be embarrassed as they play a role in public. Anticipating some of these tensions and discussing the need for support from the whole group for each student will help in allaying some of the anxieties. Sufficient time will need to be allowed for debriefing and processing students' feedback.

It is important that the students discuss and decide on the ground rules for the exercise, the time allowed for each interview, how to indicate that they need 'time out', and so on.

The success of the exercise depends to a large extent on the selection of the simulated 'client'. If possible, a specially trained person is ideal – someone who is unknown to the students and who can inject a large measure of reality into the situation. Some schools have access to simulated patients in hospital or clients in community simulations. On the other hand, effective simulations can be achieved by students working with each other, alternately playing the part of patients or client and nurse.

Although, perhaps, it is not feasible for all schools, to include domestic furniture and a typical bathroom in a practice laboratory is an excellent way to help students realize the demands of home visits or community work when the facilities always at hand in hospitals are not available.

Involving students in a simulated experience (in addition to the opportunity of practising skills) helps them to reflect on the meaning of the experience. It is a good idea to prepare questions ahead of time to stimulate students' responses and to guide their reflection, or, alternatively, you could allow time for solo reflection, then sharing this in small groups.

Finally, you could prompt students to identify their abilities in managing the frustrations during the lab exercises, in depending on resources other than the teacher's assistance and in realistic self-appraisal. These are personal learning skills which are appropriate preparation for their professional role.

Pre-clinical conference or briefing session

This includes preparation for clinical assignments with supervision to be undertaken for patients or clients in the ward, clinic or community agency.

ACTIVITY

Imagine you are preparing for a briefing session with your clinical students. What are the aims of your session?

FEEDBACK

First, it is important that clear objectives for each clinical experience be identified and shared with students and clinical staff. These objectives should refer not only to the knowledge, skills and attitudes that the students should gain but also to the level to which the student should be expected to perform.

Whether your briefing session is a brief résumé of the day's clinical assignment or a longer session of preparation of students for the individual patients or clients they will care for, your aims will include:

- discussing students' and teacher's expectations of the clinical assignment;
- encouraging students to identify their clinical learning needs;
- outlining the process of reflection-in-action, which students could use during clinical assignment;
- discussing the potential problems that could arise;
- encouraging students and fostering a colleague relationship;
- assessing whether students are adequately prepared for the work to be done;
- contracting to support a student needing assistance.

The quality of the preparation affects the value of the later reflection and exploration. Discussion in the debriefing session can then focus on, for example, whether the students' expectations were met, what actually happened during the clinical assignment and exploring what the experience means.

LEARNING ACTIVITIES IN THE BRIEFING SESSION

Carpenito and Duespohl (1985) describe briefing and debriefing as 'creative teaching tools', which should be planned together. The success of debriefing after clinical practice depends on whether the purposes of the clinical assignment have been clarified by the student and teacher in the briefing session. This means that clinical learning is not limited by the time spent and the experiences students have in the practice setting, but includes preparation for and reflection and analysis following practice.

Usually, students are involved in presenting their clinical assignments to the group followed by small-group discussion. A student-directed session involves students in identifying any concerns they may have in carrying out the assignment, discussing the preparation they have made and the reading they have done. Sometimes the teacher may need to clarify the objectives of the assignment and to advise on its feasibility for the level of the student's experience. If the student needs assistance in making links with previous learning, or in anticipating what her/his learning needs will be in the current assignment, the teacher can then raise those questions.

Briefing sessions are excellent opportunities for stimulating students to generate ideas and to suggest topics for clinical research. Obviously the level of learning and experience of your students will indicate the appropriate promptings towards the research literature that students can use.

If you have had disappointments in conducting briefing sessions, take heart. Briefing sessions are often heavy going! Students' anxieties about practice, avoiding errors and relating satisfactorily with clinical staff members and other health professionals often weigh heavily on junior students' shoulders and transfer to others in the group and to the teacher. Showing personal concern and understanding can help to reduce tension. On a practical level, agreeing with students before they begin the practice session that you will be accessible, and sharing your plan of action with them, can be immensely reassuring. Another helpful activity is to 'contract' with a student on ways you will intervene tactfully (with a prearranged sign, word or gesture) during patient or client care if the student is acting incorrectly. This measure avoids an obvious interruption and prevents embarrassment to the patient and the student.

Although a student-directed session has the potential for developing independent learning skills and in leading a group discussion, on the other hand the tendency in a group of students (depending on student-cultural mores) is to refrain from displaying their knowledge or claiming any superior skills. Handing in a written report can skirt around the problem, but for the student, opportunities to strengthen the skills of verbal communication, defending a rationale or explaining a treatment regimen and the associated nursing care are too valuable to be lost.

PRACTICE WITH SUPERVISION

CLINICAL PRACTICE SESSION – REFLECTING ON PRACTICE

Transition from classroom or simulated nursing laboratory into the real setting is the point at which many of the previously mentioned problems in clinical education arise. Some of those problems can be avoided by adequate prior planning and preparation of both students and clinical staff and some of them can be avoided by improving knowledge and practice of the clinical supervision role.

Students see clinical practice as the most important part of their programme. How can the clinical teacher maximize the opportunities for learning in clinical practice? What is the role of the teacher in a clinical practice session? Schon (1988) suggests that the teacher will be a coach – coaching students in how they use the knowledge and skills they have learnt previously and now have to apply in the real setting with real patients or clients.

Rather than being a transmitter of knowledge, the clinical teacher encourages, facilitates, and challenges the students. Through the questioning, prompting and guiding skills the students learn, step by step, to have confidence in drawing on their own store of knowledge. Moreover, as we saw in Chapter 3, clinical learning 'should build knowledge, not just use it' (Lindeman, 1989). According to Schon (1988) students learn to interpret what is happening during their experience as they reflect on the events and their actions. When this happens students are, in fact, 'building on their knowledge'.

The feedback role of the clinical teacher assumes an important place in the relationship with students. As feedback is both given to students on their performance and received from them on the clinical teacher's performance, a relationship of trust is built. Role conflict can occur between the roles of both supporter and assessor. Resolving the conflict satisfactorily depends to a large extent on the clinical teacher's ability to provide consistent, constructive and informative feedback.

To avoid the problem of students 'getting in the way' or being unwelcome in the clinical setting it is necessary to prepare the students well. Make sure that they understand the functions and organization of the ward or clinic and their place within those functions. This may have to be negotiated with clinical staff beforehand. Fothergill-Bourbonnais and Higuchi (1995) have analysed the factors involved in selecting learning experiences and have outlined the processes involved.

Clinical staff have much to offer from their experience and could be involved in the planning of objectives for clinical placements. They could also be consulted on the most appropriate tasks for the students. Regular planning or review sessions between placement supervisors and school-based teachers are a useful source of feedback to both groups on how well the curriculum is preparing the students for their jobs.

STUDENT SUPERVISION AND LEARNING ACTIVITIES

One of the biggest potential advantages of clinical education is that it provides students with the opportunity to plan their own learning, which will allow them to follow their own interests as well as achieving the stated learning objectives. To allow this to happen, the placement must give enough flexibility to allow individual student projects but also enough structure and guidance to ensure that students don't become 'lost' in the complexity of the situation. Regular sessions where groups of students and other staff can share their experiences in the placement may also be helpful. It is essential that opportunities be provided, in either simulated or low-patient-risk situations, for the students to have the freedom to observe, plan, test and evaluate their own activities. The teacher must be able to stand back and allow the students to investigate, practise and discover things for themselves. The temptation to explain everything must be resisted in favour of leaving some unknowns for the students to discover for themselves (Infante, 1985).

Clinical education offers students the opportunity to practise the roles for which they are preparing. To help them to do this students need a clear idea of their roles and their relationships with other members of the health-care team.

Effective clinical teaching suggests that:

- **Active student participation should be encouraged.** Students gain more from practising clinical or practical skills and getting feedback from the teacher than they gain from merely watching the teacher performing. One way to achieve this is role reversal, allowing the student to act as supervisor and demonstrate components of patient care, observe performance and offer constructive feedback.
- **Students should apply factual material to practical problems rather than just accumulating facts.** Teachers can help them to do this by using a problem-based approach. Start with practical problems in the clinic or ward and encourage students to analyse the problems and use their knowledge to work out possible solutions or management of the problems. Patient-centred discussions, routine ward rounds or office hand-over conferences can be organized with this aim in mind.
- **Students should be carefully supervised.** They should receive adequate feedback on their developing skills and have opportunities for progressive improvement.
- **Clinical teachers and clinical supervisors should be supportive.** Supervisors should be sensitive to the fact that students may be uncomfortable in dealing with patients or the community until they become more confident of their abilities. Clinical supervisors or teachers should avoid harsh criticism and help students to develop confidence by encouraging students to discuss their reactions to their new roles. Fishel and Johnson (1981) have described a three-way conference between student, supervisor and educator which is intended to encourage students to explore their own needs and potential and to prevent the potential problems that arise in the triangular situation in which three parties are involved but only two of the three meet on any given occasion for different purposes. Such a situation frequently gives rise to misunderstanding, discontinuity

and loss of accountability, with a resultant suboptimal learning environment for the student.

- **Clinical supervisors should be aware of – and comfortable – in a variety of roles which make up the supervisor's task.**

ACTIVITY

List the main components of the clinical supervisor's task as you know it.

FEEDBACK

An excellent analysis of the supervisor's roles has been done for teacher education (Turney *et al.*, 1983). The roles were examined by Kermode (1985) as being similar to those required for the supervision of a clinical teacher in nursing. However, there is an important difference between the application of these roles in teacher-education and in clinical nursing education. The clinical teacher is often an active partner in the clinical lesson, whereas the supervisor–teacher observes but, as a rule, does not participate in the lesson. There is more flexibility in the clinical teacher's role, as the situation may require that the teacher act as an observer so that the student's performance may be discussed later and feedback given. But more usually, the clinical teacher is a role model, an instructor and a supporter during the student's clinical assignment. Within that contextual difference, each of the facets of the role in Turney's analysis is applicable to clinical nursing education.

In brief, they can be summarized as:

- **Manager.** This role includes the successful planning and organizing of the practicum and the development of common understanding, co-operation and morale of all participants. This role builds the setting which facilitates the pursuit of all the other roles.
- **Counsellor.** This role is based on sensitivity and concern for the student as a person and as a developing nurse. It helps the student develop positive attitudes, resolve concerns, clarify behaviours and co-operate with others.
- **Instructor.** This role includes skills such as demonstrating, presenting ideas, questioning and guiding problem-solving in special tutorials and conferences.
- **Observer.** The observer role is concerned with systematically viewing and recording accurate data on the performance of the student in the clinical setting.

- **Feedback.** Through this role the supervisor conveys to the student nurse selected information arising from the observation of performance. The main purpose of this feedback is to assist the student to gauge progress and plan ways of surmounting difficulties.
- **Evaluator.** The evaluator role is concerned with making sound judgements about the level of the student's development as a nurse in relation to the aims of the clinical experience. The evaluator role, if not sensitively and supportively played, could potentially conflict with the counsellor role since the making of judgements about the student almost inevitably poses a threat to the student.

(Source: from Turney et al., 1983, p 4)

Awareness of these components of the supervisor's role assists nurse educators and supervisors to analyse their relationships with students and to discover whether there are deficiencies or imbalances which might be corrected in order to provide an optimal clinical learning experience.

Many clinical teachers would agree that the feedback role is central to clinical teaching. Casbergue (1978) has provided a classic set of guidelines for giving feedback to students in the health professions. Although the list has become well known it is worthwhile to include a brief summary in this chapter.

- Feedback should be descriptive rather than evaluative. Limit the feedback to what was said and done, or how it was accomplished (for example, the patient asked a question and you did not respond).
- Feedback should be specific rather than general.
- Feedback should focus on behaviour rather than personality.
- Feedback involves sharing of information rather than giving advice.
- Feedback should be well timed, given as near as possible to the performance.
- Feedback should be limited to the amount of information the recipient can use.
- Feedback should be directed toward behaviour the receiver can do something about.
- Feedback should be solicited rather than imposed.
- Feedback can be verified or checked by the recipient.
- Feedback can be verified or checked to determine degree of agreement from others.
- Avoid collusion in a performance which needs direct feedback.
- Feedback skills can be improved by paying attention to the consequences of the feedback.
- Constructive feedback is an important step toward authenticity.

(Source: adapted from Casbergue, 1978)

REFLECTION-IN-ACTION

The teaching skills of group discussion, facilitation, asking questions and giving informed feedback and support are necessary in clinical teaching. Schon (1988) advocates the skill of coaching for reflective teaching, particularly in reflection-in-action. It is here that the clinical teacher has a special role in standing alongside a student, in encouraging but also in acknowledging the student's ability to perform the task. Sometimes the student will follow the coach, sometimes the coach will 'jolly the student along' through humour and positive reinforcement. At other times they will both stand back and contemplate the performance from as many different angles as possible (the hall of mirrors perspective – Schon, 1988).

Boud, Keogh and Walker (1985) remind us that the reflective process is a purposeful activity, far removed from day-dreaming or putting our thoughts into idle mode. Certainly, day-dreaming is not compatible with the active nature of clinical practice. Yet the active nature of practice, the 'doing', is the context and the focus of reflective practice. How else will students discover the personal meaning of their actions than through self-reflection? Reed and Procter (1993) alert us to Schon's (1983, p 169) approach, which is not only to address issues at an individual or an interpersonal level but to include other considerations which form a framework for thinking through a particular problem.

Obviously, there is a coaching role for the clinical teacher or clinical supervisor in supporting and prompting the questions that assist reflection. It is important to note that it is not until students have a sound background knowledge in several disciplines and can process their own experience in the light of their theoretical, practical and personal knowledge that reflection-in-action can happen. In other words, students in the first years of their programme are occupied with learning the basics of the disciplines that, later on, will become the substance of reflection-in-practice. This is not to say that beginning students should not be introduced to the need to look for the personal meanings in their own actions and in the myriad of happenings around them day by day.

DEBRIEFING – REFLECTION ON PRACTICE

At the heart of the debriefing session is exploring the experience of recent clinical practice. Boud, Keogh and Walker (1985) call this 'turning experience into learning'. This involves analysis of the clinical experience, structuring reflection and deriving meaning from the experience. Obviously, these steps are very different from simply having students

nts of the clinical assignment. Ideally, capturing what the xperienced while carrying out the activities of the assignment racting meaning from the experience is the primary aim of the efing session. This does not mean that the clinical teacher avoids cking to see exactly what was done and whether the objectives of the ssignment were achieved. What it does mean is that students are made aware that the 'doing' is not the end of the learning. Briefing/debriefing sessions are part of a continuous cycle. What is discovered from the exploration of practice becomes part of the next cycle of learning.

What can the clinical teacher do to help the student 'turn experience into learning'?

There are guidelines in Matheney (1969), who points to the pre-occupation students often have with strong emotional reactions after a clinical experience. No learning will take place, Matheney advises, until students' feelings have been ventilated or resolved. However, this is not a disadvantage, as students' emotional reactions can lead to a valuable learning experience within the debriefing process.

As students realize that the knowledge they have gained from practical experience can be the building blocks of theory there needs to be 'a dialogue between what is found in practice, or in the practical situation and what is expected' (Benner, 1982). Unless the teacher is prepared for such an incident in the process of debriefing students' experiences, the opportunity for clarification may be lost. Benner adds that, without such an exploration with students, simply being in a clinical situation does not indicate that the student has 'experienced'. Posner (1985, p 19) agrees with Benner in these terms: 'We do not actually learn from experience as much as we learn from reflecting on experience'.

How can the teacher structure an exercise to assist students to reflect on experience?

A model can be very helpful in guiding the reflective process. Without a structure (derived from a model) students could easily feel that they could not 'tune in' to the abstract nature of reflection on action. Yet it is a most practical activity.

Burnard's (1987) model gives a straight forward set of steps of the cycle of experience–reflection–new experience:

- Practical experience
- Sharing of experience
- Reflection in a group on that experience

- Discussion based on the outcome of reflection; new learning is planned and developed
- Evaluation of learning and planning to apply the learning.

Another model follows the experience–reflection–outcomes pattern (Boud, 1988) and suggests that the gains from reflection on experience include the intention of some future action rather than abstract thinking. Some clarification may be required at this point (particularly with senior students) to indicate the difference between critical thinking and 'critical' reflection. The former is, of course, a necessary skill in clinical nursing and includes analysis, critique, evaluation, synthesis, so that a problem is fully investigated. Critical reflection, on the other hand is action-oriented and leads to informed committed action (Kemmis, 1985).

BRIDGING THE THEORY–PRACTICE GAP

Each decade in nursing education brings its particular focus to bear on the need to bridge the theory–practice gap. In the present decade, Andersen (1990), Perry and Jolley (1991), Gray and Pratt (1991), White and Ewan (1991), Lathlean (1992), Reed and Procter (1993) and many others point to the widening of the gap unless innovations in the organization of clinical education and in clinical learning strategies are implemented. On the other hand Cox, Hanna and Peart (1994) report a questioning of the reality of the divide between theory and practice, arguing that rather than a separation there are really recognizable linkages and 'interpenetrations'.

Organizational structures such as lecturer-practitioners, lecturer-clinicians, clinical lecturers, joint appointments and nursing development units are discussed by a number of authors in Lathlean and Vaughan (1994).

Other writers suggest several teaching–learning strategies that could bring theoretical learning and clinical learning closer together:

- clinical studies assignments
- learning diaries
- inquiry-based learning
- concept mapping
- applying social and behavioural science perspectives to clinical practice.

CLINICAL STUDIES ASSIGNMENTS

Reed and Procter (1993) include a chapter on clinical studies assignments which have been developed in the United Kingdom. Finding a clinical workbook structure too rigidly controlled, the authors developed a format consisting of a set of guidelines, allowing students the freedom to present their material in a manner of their choice.

There are three sections in the package. The first section asks students to describe their practice and aims to assist them to bring the knowledge they have gained from practice into view. 'Bringing this knowledge into view enables students to evaluate it, modify it, and question it, and to distinguish between major and minor issues in ways that may not have been available to them before.'

Section two is a review of the literature. The guidelines for students encourage them to be critical of the material they find. Students are given a summary of the types of literature and the questions to ask to be able to evaluate the validity of the material.

Section three is aimed at integrating theory with practice. The guidelines in this section are directed at relating the practice issues described in the first section with the themes extracted from the literature. Several questions assist the student by indicating the paths to follow in order to tie practice and theory together. For example:

- Does the literature have any relevance to the specific issue you have raised?
- Can you draw any conclusions from the literature which indicate possible changes in practice?
- Do you think it would be possible to implement these changes? If so describe how. If not explain why. Does your clinical practice highlight deficiencies in the literature, i.e. complexities in practice which are not considered by the literature? What are they?

The authors give a full account of their evaluation of the clinical studies assignment.

There are benefits in using a structure that helps students to affirm the value of the 'world of pragmatic and mundane issues – which is, after all, the world in which they practise and which is all too easily devalued'. Moreover, when students write from their personal perspective and reflect on their practice in a supporting environment, they gain insights which can lead to a form of action research where the problems of clinical practice are dealt with then and there.

Details of the structure of the clinical studies assignment are described by the authors, together with the descriptions of their journey through development of the methods to evaluation and continuing change.

LEARNING DIARIES

Bennett and Kingham (1993) used the concept of experiential learning to develop a learning diary. A number of curriculum objectives guided the design of the diary: for example, it should 'be student-centred, process oriented, experientially related and allow for the development of the reflective practitioner (encapsulating the theory/practice dichotomy)' (p 146). The resulting diary is semi-structured in seven sections – Introduction, A learning diary – purpose and rationale, Overview of clinical or community environment, Care in action, Analysis of your care, Bibliography, Additional notes.

The students are expected to write their experiences and their thoughts on those experiences as soon as possible. Each section of the diary gives direction to the student so that the material from reflection on the experiences can be processed systematically. It is not sufficient for the student to record a descriptive account of what happened. The experience should be analysed and related to their knowledge from a variety of sources, such as biological and social and behavioural sciences, as well as nursing theory and practice. If the student is successful in interpreting clinical practice by referring to theoretical learning, some integration of theory and practice should result. Moreover, the habits of reflection, analysis and relating experiences to theory is an important skill in understanding the significance of experiences (however everyday they may appear to be) and in preparing for independent professional practice.

INQUIRY-BASED LEARNING

This method is being developed for nursing education at the University of Hawaii. It is included here to suggest that it holds potential for reducing the practice–theory gap. Some schools of nursing have developed problem-based learning (PBL) to a sophisticated level and have shown that the integration of theory with practice has been assisted (Andersen, B., 1989; Ryan, 1989; Ryan and Little, 1989). Clinical problems are brought from the practice area and included in the programme to form 'situation improvement packages' on which students then work, eventually relating the situations back to their own clinical practice.

A comparison between PBL in medical programmes and inquiry-based learning (IBL) in a nursing programme (Feletti, 1993) limits the usefulness of the comparison, although in his analysis Feletti traces the differences in the two methods to the origin of PBL in medical programmes and the development of IBL in a nursing programme. However, within that qualification Feletti believes that IBL can be more open-ended than the PBL method.

IBL is an integrated pattern of learning experiences, beginning with the presentation of a situation which is followed by group discussion and a variety of resources. Feletti traces the method through the stages of reflection on the situation.

- **Situation.** A group of single mothers in a housing complex in an outer suburb of a large city. Resources include newspaper reports, role plays, videotaped interviews with one of the women, trigger films, discussion with a panel of appropriate community or professional members and, finally, a tutorial. Students in groups work on the question 'What is happening in this situation?'
- **Reflection.** Students may be asked to reflect on their own experiences, or any of the observations made. They may visit the suburb, interview people in the same situation, health-care condition or lifestyle.
  - Is there a problem?
  - For whom?
  - Of what dimensions?
  - Is it solvable?
  - Can things be improved?

  Students in pairs or small groups, sometimes with a tutor, meet to research the problem. This could be spread over one or more weeks, with the tutor acting as resource person, lecturer, guide, colleague or professional.
  - How am I responding?

    Students reflect on affective and self-critical aspects of feeling thinking and acting
  - Why do I see this as a problem?

    Students reflect on the situation as they see it – what prejudices, values, fundamentals do they have?
  - Do I have the tools for the job?
  - Get other information
  - Analyse and apply findings
  - What changed (in situation or in me)?
  - Where do my fundamentals come from?

    (Source: adapted from Feletti, 1993)

Feletti (1993) suggests that IBL, rather than starting with a clinical competency or a clinical situation, may 'begin with a more generic definition of inquiry skills that could suit a range of professions or disciplines, in structuring an integrated curriculum'.

CONCEPT MAPPING

Most teachers accompany their demonstrations of skills and techniques with an explanation of the theory underlying the practice. It is possible that students are so concerned about the skills and 'getting it right' that they pay less than adequate attention to the theory. Smith (1992) has used Novak and Gowin's (1984) method of concept mapping and the Vee heuristic to emphasize the influence of theory on each step of a nursing skill. The example Smith gives starts with a focus question for students: 'How can a nurse begin mobilizing a patient safely?' 'Dangling the immobilized patient' is the nursing event for which students then identify the appropriate theoretical principles (e.g. from biological, social and behavioural sciences and nursing theory). The benefits and hazards of dangling from a nursing knowledge and value perspective are included and, finally, a set of concepts is identified.

The concepts (homoeostasis, vasodilation, dangle, blood pooling, orthostatic hypertension) are then plotted so that the linkages between the action of dangling and its underlying theory are clear. Smith claims that mapping can clarify students' misconceptions before any new learning takes place. Also, students often find that in comparison with 'doing' nursing taking time to understand the theory is frustrating. Smith has found that the concrete nature of the concept mapping and Vee heuristic strategy 'is a powerful way to link theory and practice for nursing curricula' (Smith, 1992).

VIDEOTAPED DEMONSTRATIONS OF APPLYING SOCIAL AND
BEHAVIOURAL SCIENCE PERSPECTIVES TO CLINICAL PRACTICE

With the advent of the development of 14 nursing courses within the higher education system of Australia in the late 1980s the spotlight was turned on curriculum developers. A long-awaited opportunity to identify a distinctively Australian pattern of learning and to put it in to practice was grasped enthusiastically. A study commissioned by the Bicentennial Committee to Review Australian Tertiary Studies in Education (CRASTE) found 'a profession "remaking" itself, in the act of transformation to an academic discipline. It also encountered an emerging body of nursing knowledge, sensitive to the complexities of Australian society and its systems of health-care delivery' (Cottier, 1986, p 156).

In the newly developed courses many course objectives were framed in such a way as to indicate high expectations of successful application of theory to practice: for example, 'be able to apply relevant theoretical concepts and principles in the performance of selected nursing care activities for individuals across the age continuum and in different disorder categories'; or 'ability to use understanding (of the different theories of human development through the lifespan) and awareness as the base for the development of professional competency which can be applied in a wide range of cultural contexts'.

What could clinical teachers do? The need was to assist students to draw on the material they received from the theoretical programme and to guide them through clinical problems so that they could see how and where to apply concepts from theory.

Perry (1991) notes that 'health and illness always involve psychological and physical causes and effects. Patients are thinking and reasoning individuals and not simply bedridden or ambulatory cases!'

The perceived relevance of theory to practical nursing was not such a problem for students in the area of biomedical science, since there is a long tradition of working within a biomedical model. On the other hand, the increases in the theoretical content of the social and behavioural sciences taught by teachers who were knowledgeable in their disciplines but who were without clinical knowledge or experience resulted in serious theory–practice gaps.

A grant to develop a resource project was received by the authors from CRASTE. A series of videotaped critical incidents was filmed to portray how clinical teachers guide their students in dealing with problems which cannot be resolved by an appeal to the biological base of the patient's illness. Nor can the student deal with the social and behavioural aspects alone: she/he must assess the influence of the physical and physiological component at the same time. In the critical incidents portrayed on the tapes the student deals with the implications of the physical condition as well as trying to understand the behaviour before deciding how to proceed.

To fulfil the requirements of the grant the project focused on including Australian material into tertiary studies. Accordingly, five major issues impinging on health care in Australia were selected (Table 5.1) although the issues are not exclusive to one country and have wider application. The issues were:

- the lifestyle differences that create barriers between Australian nurses and patients or clients;
- child sexual abuse, the family and the health-care system;
- the well but frail elderly needing care;
- Aboriginal people admitted to hospital;
- the induction of tertiary students into the health-care system and the nursing profession.

Table 5.1 Framework of the project (source: White *et al.*, 1988)

Focus	Social behavioural perspectives	Clinical teaching skills
Lifestyle	Symbolic interaction theory	Counselling technique
Aboriginal health	Cultural communication	Partnership in learning
Child sexual abuse	Systems theory	Social networking
Professional socialization	Role theory	Coordinator of learning
Age	Stereotyping	Life review strategy

Example of a videotaped critical incident

An example of a debriefing session from the tape *Critical Incidents in Clinical Teaching* (1988) follows.

The students are attached to a paediatric ward for their clinical placement. One of the children, Michelle, confided in a student (Sue) that she has been sexually abused by her father. The clinical teacher (CT) is responding to Sue's question, 'What should I do?'

The clinical teacher counsels Sue and explains that the authorities have to be notified of child sexual abuse as it is a legal requirement in that State. The student has difficulty in realizing the nature of her role in caring for Michelle. The clinical teacher prompts the student to think about the needs of her patient. The social and behavioural perspective is systems theory and networking.

The clinical teaching prompts, which appear as superscripts on the screen, are:

- Raising implications
- Questioning limits
- Applying theory
- Encouraging reflection.

CT: What are Michelle's most important needs at the moment?
Sue: To be safe, to be protected, to be loved – I guess to know that I'm here to help her.
CT: How might you tell her that?
Sue: I could just stay with her; I could let her know that I care about her.
CT: Is there anything else you need to tell her?
Sue: No – I don't think so. Oh yes, we should tell her that I've notified the authorities.– that'll be hard for her. Isn't that breaking confidentiality?
Raising implications
CT: Yes, that's true, but you had already told me that you made that decision because you were worried about Michelle and if

you don't follow through with that, then Michelle may not get the care she needs.

Sue: So, I have to weigh up what's the most important thing – to keep confidentiality because that's a most important personal thing, or break confidentiality again so that Michelle gets the help she needs.

CT: Before we go any further, let's look at that networking you were doing before. There is a referral system for Michelle's problem, and remember that we still don't actually know what happened to her.

Sue: How will we find out?

CT: How do you think we'd go about that?

Sue: Well, Michelle thinks she's shared the information with me only. So it's really between Michelle and myself, isn't it?

Questioning limits

CT: Do you mean you want to take the responsibility yourself?

Sue: No.

CT: So what do you think is best for Michelle?

Sue: To get help from people who care about her.

CT: And who might that be?

Sue: I guess the experts in this sort of thing.

CT: Yes, if you think back to what we were saying about health care as being part of a whole system of linkages – in this case Michelle needs expert help and the way we do that is by notification of the problem.

Sue: Well, I still want to help, too.

CT: Well, of course, but let's take a moment to sort out where we are.

Applying theory

(The clinical teacher draws a circle on a white board in the office.)

CT: Let's say this is Michelle, and this represents you (draws another circle). Is there anyone else involved in this?

Sue: The family (draws another circle).

CT: Is there anything else that will help you to understand the problem?

Sue: No, I don't think so.

CT: Well, is it just a problem in the relationship between Michelle and her father?

Sue: (pauses) No, it must be more than that because the authorities have to be notified.

Encouraging reflection

CT: OK. So does that mean that it involves society as a whole?

Sue: (Long pause) I guess so, but I don't really know – I'm not really sure (struggling, appears troubled).

CT: Well, what do you think? (draws a large circle to enclose all smaller circles).

Sue: I guess so.

CT: Well, problems like these can't be left to the two parties to work out between themselves; they need to be dealt with by mechanisms that society as a whole has put into place and Michelle's problem needs to be seen in that broader context.

In the group debriefing session the next day the clinical teacher turns the session over to Sue for her to explain how she had to learn to deal with the complexities of a social problem and an ethical dilemma, and how a theoretical perspective helped her to understand her nursing actions and her role.

One could argue that the context of the client is not so important in understanding and applying concepts from the biological sciences, since they may be applied universally and are not, as a rule, culture-dependent. Diagnosing and meeting the 'situationally-derived needs' (Woolridge, Skipper and Leonard, 1968, p 11) of the patient or client is a major nursing responsibility, making knowledge and application of social and behavioural science perspectives an essential component of clinical nursing practice.

PLANNING CLINICAL LEARNING

We have covered quite a number of important points in planning and carrying out effective clinical learning experiences. The next activity asks you to reflect on what we have covered and to integrate it into a plan that you would be able to use in your own particular situation.

ACTIVITY

Make a checklist which you can use to help you in planning clinical learning for students that you teach.

FEEDBACK

Clinical learning should involve learning by doing. It is a difficult but valuable experience which should not be wasted on teaching that could take place just as well in the classroom. Adequate preparation of students, supervisors and the other people who are part of the clinical setting is essential if learning by doing is to occur in the clinical placement. Given this *sine qua non* for clinical teaching and learning, the following points may be helpful reminders when planning clinical placements for your students.

Define goals for clinical learning

Have you decided whether you want your students to:

- learn psychomotor skills;
- deal with real problems;
- understand the realities of the nurse's job;
- develop attitudes;
- develop communication skills;
- learn to plan patient care;

or

- achieve all of these objectives?

Remember, each clinical experience must be accompanied by a clear statement about what students are expected to achieve during that experience.

Plan clinical experience

Are you going to involve the clinical staff and supervisors in planning objectives and methods?

What experiences will you provide in the classroom to prepare students for the real situation when they enter the clinical placement?

Will clinical staff and supervisors be trained in effective supervision?

Plan clinical programme

Will you:

- involve patients and/or community groups in the teaching?
- ensure that students' roles and tasks are explicit and understood?
- encourage students to perform real tasks and use their own judgement?
- use a problem-based approach that allows students to discover appropriate strategies or plan interventions?
- provide adequate supervision and feedback on performance?
- encourage students to take responsibility for their own learning?

- devise ways to assess student performance 'on the job' and to provide progressive feedback as an integral part of learning?
- allow adequate opportunities for students to reflect on their experience?
- keep clinical staff informed of the students' programme?

Teaching and learning in the workplace

6

INTRODUCTION

Most teachers in nursing are concerned with guiding students through the undergraduate course, so that by graduation they will be prepared to function as professional nurses. Throughout this book the focus is on achieving this goal through well chosen content and learning experiences and specially designed teaching/learning sequences in both classroom and clinical practice. What happens to those graduates during their introduction into the workplace as employees? As members of a team? As professionals implementing and applying knowledge compiled during the course and now used in the workplace?

In this chapter we will focus on registered nurses (RNs) as learners in the context of practice (new graduate, post-registration student, re-entry after years of absence, RN staff new to an area or to a different institution or to a change in routine) and their teachers, not as clinical teachers but as 'workplace teachers'. There are obvious differences between the approaches, methods and programme designs adopted by workplace teachers responsible for the further learning of graduates and clinical teachers responsible for undergraduate teaching. We will pursue these differences and their implications for teaching and learning.

Certainly the period of change represents an important transition for all RNs proceeding from one stage of professional learning to the next. What is the nature of teaching and learning in this transition context? The question is urgent for new graduates, but is also relevant to RNs returning to practice through a re-entry programme, transition of experienced professional staff new to a different and/or unfamiliar area of practice, professional staff changing from one institution to another, or staff during periods of change, e.g. changes in an established routine, the introduction and use of new complex equipment and the mastering of information technology.

When you finish this chapter you should be able to design learning programmes for professional staff, drawing on learning principles and approaches and exploring your role as it changes from teaching undergraduate students to teaching postgraduate registered nurses.

WORKPLACE LEARNING

Clinical teachers have accepted the responsibility of preparing students for professional practice, but the context of their responsibilities is the academic course and the philosophy and policies are those of the university or college. Graduates are no longer part of that undergraduate context, but have moved into another. Now, the post-registration context is occupational, and it is the hospital, clinic or community philosophy and policy, with the associated work ethic, established communication channels and administrative power and processes.

The workplace and workplace learning has received increased attention in recent years following the questioning of its often mechanistic character by well known authors such as Knowles (1975). Learning in the workplace departs from the paradigms of training ('short-term activities that emphasize practical skills immediately applicable to a job') and education ('longer-term courses that develop generic knowledge, skills and abilities rather than job-related competencies') (Marsick, 1987, p 3).

> Training and education are delivery systems. By contrast, learning is the way in which individuals or groups acquire, interpret, reorganize, change or assimilate a related cluster of information, skills and feelings. It is also primary to the way in which people construct meaning in their personal and shared organizational lives. Learning takes place through daily interaction and experience within the organization, whether or not it has been structured by trainers. It is often self-directed and self-monitored and includes informal modes such as coaching, mentoring and working groups focused around a specific task.
>
> *(Source: Marsick, 1987, p 4)*

The informal learning described by Marsick as central to learning in the workplace will have been experienced by most health professionals. By 'daily interaction and experience' new graduates observe the actions, gestures, language and working styles of the more experienced. What they are learning through self-direction and self-monitoring is as personal as it is imperceptible, but the result for neophytes is the difference between acceptance by the work group or alienation until socialization has been achieved.

What guidelines are there to assist in learning and teaching in the workplace?

Mezirow (1985) has offered a set of principles of learning in the workplace which Marsick has adapted. How appropriate are they for the contexts in which nurses work and learn?

ACTIVITY

Think about your current experience of learning in your present workplace, either as a learner or as a teacher. Which of the following principles of learning are you able to implement? Why are you unable to implement them all?

Learners in the workplace:

- participate freely and fully in collaborative problem-solving;
- are encouraged to take different perspectives, attitudes and roles *vis-à-vis* their work;
- can ask questions, receive accurate and considerate feedback, and reflect on themselves;
- can share progressively in decision-making;
- can think critically and reflectively; can question what is taken for granted including organizational norms, established ways of thinking and belief systems;
- can experiment without serious consequences;
- can make inferences from daily activities that enable them to learn how to learn and to solve long-range problems;
- have a climate of mutual respect for one another's self-worth;
- can be free to pursue self-directed learning and are encouraged to become increasingly empowered *vis-à-vis* their work;
- learn through mentoring, coaching and small-group work.

(Source: adapted from Mezirow by Marsick, 1987, p 200)

FEEDBACK

No doubt your reasons for being unable to implement some of the above principles are based on the nature of health-care institutions and agencies that emphasize safe, quality care. For example, being able to experiment with a change of routine may be possible, since nurses can be autonomous in introducing nursing-care processes. On the other hand, changes or experiments with treatments need to be approved by research and ethics committees, as well as management. The freedom to question may be another principle which may not always be possible to implement, nor is receiving considerate, informed feedback so that self-reflection can follow. Other principles, such as a climate of mutual respect, thinking critically and reflectively, learning how to learn and pursuing self-directed learning, can be implemented by individuals and by so doing the larger group is also influenced.

In summary, if a learning environment can be established in the workplace most of the principles of learning can be implemented.

CHARACTERISTICS OF A WORKPLACE LEARNING ENVIRONMENT

ACTIVITY

Imagine you have been given the opportunity for designing a learning environment for your department or work group. What are the major considerations you would include?

FEEDBACK

It is helpful to again refer to Marsick's (1987) work and below is a set of characteristics of a workplace learning environment. There is an interesting paradox here. Such is the nature of reflective and critically reflective workplace learning espoused by Marsick, that a 'cook-book recipe' list for its implementation seems directly opposite to the principles stated above. Nevertheless, Marsick provides a set of characteristics of a workplace learning environment. How many of these characteristics are possible for guiding workplace learning in your environment?

- Reflection on practice and in learning that is at times critical
- Full and free dialogue leading to conscious creation and examination of goals, norms and values
- Concern for setting the problem as well as solving it
- Public experimentation and inquiry leading to fresh approaches to action

- Reliance on team group learning for both individual and collective processes
- Enhancement of self-esteem, self-discovery and self-directedness
- Acknowledgment of importance of whole person, including feelings and emotions, in learning
- Internal, rather than external, motivation characterized by autonomy and empowerment of individuals to go beyond self-imposed internal limits or externally imposed organizational constraints
- Continuous informal learning on the job fostered through networks of learning relationships (coaching, mentoring) and supplemented appropriately by formal training.

(Source: Marsick, 1987, p 203)

Creating a learning environment in a health-care workplace with its goals, values, norms, roles and power and authority hierarchies obviously, by its very nature, needs to be a collaborative and co-operative development between education and administration.

ACTIVITY

One of the ways the workplace teacher can implement a learning environment for new graduates is to consider their problems as they first arrive on the job. Read the following account of a new graduate's first day. Your own experience as a new registered nurse in beginning professional practice may have been similar to the first day described below. Identify the major problems in such an experience and suggest ways they can be overcome.

I arrive on the ward at 7 am sharp, shaking. Hospitals have a very distinct smell. I try to imagine facing that smell every morning for the rest of my working life. I sit with four other Registered Nurses in the ward tea-room, waiting for the morning report. I am embarrassed about my new regulation nursing shoes. We sit, quietly and professionally sipping coffee. My hands begin to sweat.

An RN walks in to give her report. I pick up my pen to record important points about each patient, and wonder what is important and what is not. I should know, but I feel as though I've forgotten everything I've learnt. The RN and others to follow speak very quickly and in initials. I have no idea what they all stand for and have neither the time nor the courage to ask.

The report ends and I am allocated six patients to look after. I am not sure what is wrong with any of them. I am sure, however, that they are all sick and, for the next 8 hours, my responsibility. I introduce myself to them and worry that they can see how frightened I am.

My first task is to give all these pained faces their morning medications. There seem to be thousands of tablets and I am only almost sure of the purpose of half of them. A patient asks me what a tablet is for. Oh dear! I should know. I have to look it up. I feel embarrassed and stupid.

A patient must now be prepared for theatre immediately. I haven't finished the pills. The porters are here to take the patient. I quickly get the patient ready, disturbed by the fear on his face, and regret not having the time to comfort him. Suddenly I am rushing down corridors beside the trolley to theatres. I wish we could slow down. The theatres look like something from a science fiction movie and the staff like aliens.

I fly back to the ward to find the pill trolley missing – they will now have to wait. I take all their observations, keeping one eye open for the pill trolley. One patient's blood pressure is way too high. The wound of a man that I sent to the shower has started to bleed and two ladies want pans now! I seem to be running in circles. Another patient to theatre, one with chest pain, have to make the beds.

Lunch time goes past like a flash and I return to the ward in time to receive a patient back from theatre with more drips and drains than I have ever seen before. Dressings to do, more pills . . . the NUM grabs me and says, 'Give a hand-over, write your reports and go home'.

I think about all the things that still have to be done and pray I haven't missed something crucial, I am confused, my feet hurt and I am exhausted, I am not sure I am cut out for all this. I leave the hospital in a daze.

(Source: Scott and Underwood, 1991)

FEEDBACK

First days as a registered nurse can be memorable. For some, the change in status, uniform and job is a long awaited reward; for others, poised uncertainly on the threshold of new responsibilities, the prospect is daunting. For many it is the first experience of employment; they have been students most of their lives. The change from dependence on a well known system to independence in an unfamiliar context generates fear as well as eager anticipation. Will there be acceptance by experienced RNs? Will there be encouragement and assistance if needed? Will patients or clients detect and understand both the anxiety and eagerness to succeed?

The major problems experienced to some degree by most new graduates are:

- **Dependence on trial-and-error learning.** Being left to 'sink or swim', with its associated stresses and traumas, leads, not surprisingly, to frustrations and disappointments and eventually to resignations from the workplace. While some educators recommend a degree of anxiety as a motivator for learning, in the clinical field it is not only the learner who is vulnerable but the patients or clients who may be affected by the anxiety of a new graduate. Without collegial support to empower the new graduate and to build confidence the transition period becomes a period of self-doubt and feelings that success in nursing will be unachievable.
- **Unfamiliar language.** One of the hurdles to be overcome for new graduates is the feeling of being on the 'outer', not yet accepted by co-workers. The symbols, customs and shared meanings that are a part of the professional culture are a source of confusion and a barrier to becoming accepted. There is an overriding desire to communicate and to understand the communication of others. Until the barrier of the 'in' language has been overcome, new graduates feel at a loss to understand what is meant by the abbreviations and jargon terminology.
- **Unfamiliar report requirements.** Although fresh from the undergraduate course new graduates are astonished that their knowledge seems irrelevant to the information about patients and clients and their treatments described in duty reports. Instead of the rejection they expected because of their 'book knowledge' they find that the knowledge shared at report hand-over might as well be in a foreign language, which indeed it is, to them. To ask for translation is to admit to an embarrassing ignorance.

- **Contrast between beliefs and values of university and work settings.** For new graduates with no prior experience of employment the difference between the comparative freedom of university life and the prescriptive demands of work life may come as a shock. A new world confronts them as they come face to face with 'the realization . . . that they must conform to the established procedures and practices of the organization far more than they had anticipated' (Stoner, Collins and Yetton, 1985, p 683).
- **Unrealistic expectations of their own performance.** Making judgements about their performance in comparison with experienced RNs is a common source of frustration during the transition period. 'They enter a transitional state of normlessness in which they are neither student nor proficient RN. This temporary state increases their anxiety and may result in resignations as a means of escaping from a seemingly unbearable situation' (Andersen, S. L., 1989, p 23).
- **Priority setting among tasks and clients.** Separating urgent and non-urgent problems is a sophisticated activity. Not all experienced RNs are necessarily skilled in responding to priorities. New graduates are understandably confused when decisions are needed based on clinical experience rather than subject knowledge. Moreover, Kramer (1985, p 902) believes that the 'priority problem' is one of values. 'The problem is that the student's value system is different from the dominant and prevailing value system at work.'
- **Transition from student role to staff nurse role.** Moving to a staff nurse role and taking responsibility for the management of patient care throws up stark disparities between the two roles, leading to professional and personal conflicts (McGrath and Princeton, 1987). Kramer (1985) claims that the nursing service is often inconsistent and unclear about the role of staff nurse that the new graduate should play.
- **Difficulty in asking for help when needed for fear of appearing inadequate.** The 'hidden curriculum' during the transition period is that asking for help is confirmation of incompetence and dependence. Once these labels have been attached they are likely to stay and travel with the graduate to other work areas.

What can the workplace teacher do? How can new graduates be assisted to overcome these problems? How can the principles of learning in the workplace and a positive learning environment help during the transition period?

WORKPLACE TEACHING – ASSISTING TRANSITION IN THE WORKPLACE

The transition from one environment to another can be facilitated through:

- preceptorships;
- an orientation programme.

PRECEPTORSHIPS

In some institutions, preceptors are assigned to each new graduate to provide support and guidance and to help them in negotiating the first weeks (or months) of their appointments. New graduates find that preceptors, who are selected because they are familiar with the organization, the institution and the care of patients or clients, are able to offer help in settling into the responsibilities and demands of a new workplace. However, preceptors (with special time to assist new graduates) are not always available. Clinical staff, ward sisters and clinical staff specialists may then be responsible for assisting new graduates.

The literature on preceptorship in nursing dates from 1974, as a response to Kramer's (1974) description of reality shock. During the two decades since its introduction the concept of preceptorship has had many interpretations. Henry and Ensunsa (1991, p 52) report that preceptors have been used for both student nurses and nurse orientees and that 'the preceptor serves three important functions whether precepting a student nurse or a nurse orientee: clinical instructor, professional role-model and resource'.

In the Australian context, Mascord (1992) distinguishes between preceptors and clinical teachers. The main role of the former is the care of patients or clients. The preceptorship role is added in order to assist new people into a new work situation, to help them find their way around and 'to understand the employing institution's values and goals'. In addition, the preceptor assists new graduates to 'apply theory to practice with a particular group of patients/clients, to set priorities, organize and evaluate their own patient care and to work as an independent member of the team as soon as possible' (p 1). The point is made that their responsibility for a full clinical load as an employee of the health-care institution is different from the clinical teacher, who is responsible for the education of students during their undergraduate course. The preceptor is, therefore, a workplace teacher in every sense of the word.

Armitage and Burnard (1991) examined the concepts of preceptor and mentor and found that while there were similarities in some of the activities, there were clear differences in the role. 'The mentor role seems to be more about "looking after" the learner nurse, whilst the preceptor role seems to be more concerned with enhancing clinical competence through direct role-modelling' (p 228). Reed and Procter (1993) do not mention preceptors but agree that the role of mentor requires clarification, particularly in respect of their activities in post-registration programmes.

Although the terminology and descriptions may differ from country to country and in various institutions, there is a common aim to assist learning in the workplace, be it the new graduate, the returning registered nurse, the in-service or staff development participant or the post-registration student.

ORIENTATION

New graduates want to succeed. They want to know what indicates success in their work environment and they want to get there as quickly as possible. They also want to know who is influential in their new workplace; who will help, who can be asked questions without fear of intimidation. They are anxious to do the 'right' thing and want to know what to do if they make a mistake.

How often are these points addressed in orientation? More often the orientation is completed as quickly as possible because of the demands of a busy ward, clinic or community agency. Yet new graduates need opportunities for open discussion about the characteristics of the work and the expectations of superiors. When this occurs in an atmosphere that demonstrates that they are welcome and that their individual qualities, needs and qualifications are accepted, new graduates feel valued.

ACTIVITY

Imagine you are to conduct an orientation programme for new graduates in your institution. Based on the problems of new graduates discussed above, and the principles of workplace learning, make a list of aims for such a programme.

FEEDBACK

Your selection of aims will depend on the possibilities and the constraints of your organization. Above all, the aims should be realistic and attainable. Basically the overall aim is to assist new graduates to achieve a smooth transition into the workplace while providing support and encouragement, recognizing the individual worth and contribution each can make. In addition an orientation programme seeks to assist new graduates to:

- resolve the separation/termination from nursing school;
- learn to appraise their own performance realistically;
- share their concerns without fear of reprisals;
- reduce the dissonance between theory and practice;
- develop an understanding of the occupational context;
- identify their role-relations with members of nursing and other health profession staff.

(Adapted from Andersen, S. L., 1989)

Resolving the separation/termination from nursing school

To some extent the change of uniform, including a graduation badge, is a visual indicator of a changed status from student to professional nurse. Socialization into the professional culture requires a special social interaction of new graduates and experienced RNs where there are reciprocal expectations.

Kramer (1974) described the transition as 'reality shock' and recommended certain changes to the undergraduate course to reduce the distance between an idealistic view of nursing from the perspective of academia and the everyday realities of health care in the context of pressures from bureaucracy. One decade later Kramer (1985) asked why reality shock continued. Her conclusion was that it had to. 'Reality shock is the overt manifestation of a deep underlying conflict – a conflict at the very essence of nursing' (p 891). Kramer explains that reality shock continues for three main reasons:

- the nature of service and education goals;
- nurse education's abdication of responsibility;
- unclear and unrealistic goals of nursing service.

Benner redefines 'reality shock' as 'that uncomfortable process of gaining experiential learning that cannot be conveyed by formal models, formal theories, or forecasts about what a situation will be like' (Benner, 1984, p 188). Informal learning in the workplace is therefore as important as guidance during early work experiences and can be encouraged by recognizing the value of self-pacing, by supportive relationships and by allowing for individual differences in early work achievements.

Learning to appraise their own performance realistically

Benner (1984) questioned the discrepancy between beginner nurse, nursing education and nursing service performance expectations as 'a crisis in confidence, rather than in ability'. When nursing service personnel were asked to appraise actual performance of a particular new nurse (rather than their ideal expectations of new nurses in general) the appraisal of performance was higher (Benner, 1984, p 188). Benner explains the differences in the appraisals and expectations of new graduates by nursing service and nursing education as negative stereotyping of the new graduate by nursing service persons and a basic difference between nursing service and nursing education in perception and understanding of skilled performance (p 189).

Sharing concerns without fear of reprisals

Smythe (1984) and S. L. Andersen (1989) emphasize the value of support systems in assisting nurses to cope with stress. Smythe advocates social networks while Andersen describes the role of a 'nurse advocate' who is not involved in clinical orientation of new graduates and is separate from a preceptor or other clinical staff. The nurse advocate is familiar with the formal and informal networks of the institution as well as providing a forum for sharing of concerns, the exploration of stressors and the role-playing of behaviours to enhance professional effectiveness in the realm of assertiveness and decision-making (Andersen, S. L., 1989).

Reducing dissonance between theory and practice

Learning shifts from a subject base to a performance base (Lickman, Simms and Green, 1993, p 212). This does not mean that knowledge acquired during the course is irrelevant to performance. In fact, the preparation of 'knowledgeable doers' is the underlying purpose of new courses in the United Kingdom (Perry and Jolley, 1991). The intent is not so much to integrate what has been acquired in subjects with what is required in performance, but to plan learning during the course so that knowing and doing are forged together, firmly linked and purposeful, enabling practitioners to learn and use knowledge in the context of performance.

Developing an understanding of the occupational context

Early work experiences leave an indelible impression and play a critical role in the way new graduates perceive the employing body's expectations of them and how the organization attempts to meet the graduate's expectations (Stoner, Collins and Yetton, 1985). Careful counselling, assisting graduates to identify their expectations and clarifying any misconceptions, is an essential role for the preceptor. One of the challenges thrown out to students during the undergraduate course is that they are expected to be change agents. There is no doubt that the profession sorely needs them, and graduates may be keen to adopt that role. Confronted by the realization of the status of employees in a large organization, the role of change agent for the new graduate becomes eclipsed by the need to conform to established procedures and practices far more than they had anticipated (Stoner, Collins and Yetton, 1985).

There are shocks for new graduates schooled in the philosophy of personalized, individualized care when the full force of modern health-care cost-conscious methods is met. 'The language used to discuss hospital services is the language of the market place. Patient care is now the hospital product and DRGs allow hospitals to select those products to which they can devote their energies and resources most productively' (Biscoe, 1989, p 111). If quality of care is emphasized and patient care is not depersonalized, health-care services are enhanced and the patient benefits. New graduates may need help from skilled staff to understand the context in which they will implement individualized care. Furthermore, new graduates may carry the ideologies of the change agent role into their first work experiences, expecting to see that experienced practitioners are enacting the role and achieving success in 'changing the system'. While there is broad allegiance by the profession for the policy of positive influence and inclusion of nurses in forums responsible for setting health-care goals, skilled experienced clinicians as well as new graduates need an enlightened understanding of 'the system' and the society in which it functions (Biscoe, 1989).

Identifying role relationships with nursing and other health professional staff

There are rewards for clinical staff willing to share with new graduates the skills they have developed. Certainly, the rewards also come with considerable cost. Recognition of the expertise of skilled practitioners is often overlooked in the pressure of heavy workloads and rising bed occupancy rates. While tensions may arise in busy workplaces and slow new workers can be an added cause of frustration, skilled staff are in even more demand to provide stability and consistency in what seems, to the uninitiated, a whirling world of change.

ACTIVITY

Whatever form the orientation programme takes, and regardless of its length, there are several essentials which should be included to provide new graduates with a sense that they are welcome and that their ideas and comments are valuable. Make a list of the essentials you would try to include.

FEEDBACK

Allow time in your orientation programme for:

- inviting new graduates to suggest topics important to them to be included in the programme;
- recognizing each new graduate individually, getting to know their background, interests and needs for orientation, and for their clinical and nursing careers;
- discussing the experience of being a new graduate in the department and institution (hospital, clinic, community agency);
- encouraging reflection on their experiences during the orientation and following experiences;
- promoting a feeling of identification with the occupational setting;
- providing protocols and work schedules appropriate to the experience and competencies of the new graduates;
- introducing the philosophy and objectives of the department, its organizational structure and functions, communication channels and the context of the department within the total institution;
- providing workshops on clinical responsibilities and quality assurance principles, documentation and reporting procedures and staff appraisal methods and principles;
- discussing legal and ethical principles relevant to the department and clinical practice;
- identifying personnel of the department and the wider institution, and their roles, availability of and access to support and advisory personnel;
- indicating the programmes of ongoing learning within the department;

- giving the location of equipment and resources;
- demonstrating equipment and special methods used in the department, if required, and giving the rationale for their use;
- including clinical staff in the orientation programme.

POST-REGISTRATION EDUCATION

As undergraduate nurse education takes its place in the context of higher education in most countries, the question of appropriate post-registration education becomes a prominent debating point amongst nursing leaders. Reed and Procter, for example, say that 'to have a situation where a nurse undergoes a dynamic and creative initial education programme, and then stops at the moment of qualification, is to do an injustice to practitioners' (1993, p 183). Future developments for post-registration education and practice that aim to support a level of practice include an 'advanced practitioner' (p 187). Perry and Jolley (1991) point to the preparation of 'knowledgeable practitioners' who will exercise skills of critical analysis, critical reflection and decision-making.

There is a challenge for teachers in planning post-registration education so that the experience and knowledge of students is recognized (Eason and Corbett, 1991). If the course is planned as mainly academic, it is likely that experienced practitioners will undervalue their clinical knowledge and experience as they are confronted by theoretical approaches of an academic course. 'The post-registration students' problem is not that "they do not know what they need to know", more that "they do not know what they **do** know" (Reed and Procter, 1993, p 40). As we have seen, if the course centres on technical and mechanistic skills, the personal growth of individual RNs could be disregarded.

ACTIVITY

Your experience as a teacher of nursing students has, most probably, been predominantly in teaching either undergraduate or postgraduate nurses. On the other hand, you may be teaching both groups and the differences required may be well known to you. Let's clarify the differences by making a comparison between the clinical teacher in undergraduate programmes and the workplace teacher in a health-care institution.

First, make a list of the factors where the differences in approach will be most apparent. Then compare how each factor affects the clinical teacher and the workplace teacher.

FEEDBACK

The major differences (Table 6.1) are in:

- the status of students;
- the relation of teacher with students;
- the roles of teachers;
- the context in which teaching is practised;
- the culture of the learner's environment;
- the focus of the teacher;
- the learning environment;
- relations with patients or clients.

Table 6.1   Comparisons between clinical teachers and workplace teachers

	Clinical teacher	Workplace teacher
Status of students	Undergraduate	Professional members of staff
Relation with students	Authority through academic role	Equal professionals, both qualified, with professional autonomy
Roles	Teachers, facilitators, assessors	Preceptors, mentors, supervisors clinical specialist facilitators, appraisers
Context	Academic institution and clinical placements	Health-care institution
Culture	Student School	Professional occupation
Focus	Assisting learning in preparation for practice	Assisting performance and job-related competencies and career plans
Learning environment	Student groups, one to one	Work team
Relation with students in clinical practice	Students dependent Supervised practice	Students independent Usually unsupervised practice

IMPLICATIONS FOR TEACHING IN POST-REGISTRATION PROGRAMMES

ACTIVITY

Post-registration learners come to the workplace from re-entry courses, in-service, or post-registration courses (leading to an award) with a variety of approaches they have developed from former education and from life experiences. Think of your own post-registration learning and identify some of the needs you and your colleagues had in that experience.

FEEDBACK

Needs as learners

As mature learners, post-registration students are often subject to stressors because of their motivation to succeed. The personal standard of their own performance is often set at a much higher level than their teachers set for them. As a result, the experience of returning to learning can be difficult, especially for sensitive individuals who assume that an atmosphere of competition will naturally occur in the group. Although this is probably a misconception, earlier unpleasant memories of less-than-happy learning experiences may persist.

Again, because of their maturity and life situations, they may be facing similar problems to those their patients and clients are undergoing, learning, for example, how to assist their patients or clients through developmental crises such as facing decisions about marriage and childbearing and -rearing, caring for elderly parents and providing support for family members who may be disabled. As they learn how to assist, their own needs for assistance in comparable situations may become more apparent and pressing.

Certainly, personal and family responsibilities of post-registration students are likely to be heavier than those of high-school leavers in undergraduate programmes. Some courses carry expensive course fees and financial pressures can place additional stress on a learner who also has family responsibilities.

Registered nurses re-entering professional nursing after being professionally inactive do so for reasons of decreasing family responsibilities, economic necessity (finding a regular income necessary through divorce and/or solo parenting), and the general devaluing of housekeeping and childrearing as a legitimate role in society. 'The decrease in self-image and status emanating from this role has brought many women to re-consider re-activating their professional nursing role' (Hengstberger-Sims, 1987).

Many registered nurses in Hengstberger-Sims's study left the profession during early work experiences, finding the pressure of work and inadequate staffing levels stressful. The uncongenial and unsuitable work hours, inadequate salary and impoverished status of nursing led to professional disillusionment. Their decision to re-enter and gain access to employment via a refresher course was chosen rather than the more threatening direct re-entry by on-the-job retraining. Some of the improvements they expected to see may not have materialized. Studying the complexities of modern health-care systems either increases their understanding of the difficulties or reinforces their previous dissatisfaction.

Most re-entry courses are planned on the assumption that students want to upgrade their knowledge and skills. Certainly, having the confidence to perform successfully depends on being able to meet the standards of competency demanded. However, there are other aspects that post-registration students find worrying and are in need of some discussion and support. Sweetwood (1986) discovered that ethical questions about new technology, new roles for nurses and new legislation were a central concern. Post-registration students require orientation sessions that recognize the possibility of wide individual differences as well as a common reaction to the strangeness and newness of a new role and a new workplace.

Needs as professionals

Post-registration students often reject the notion of professional resocialization as they perceive that they are already professionals. In addition, learning new roles and role relationships often arouses strong feelings. The student's personal and professional identity can be threatened. Respect for their experience and knowledge is needed and recognition of the skill of 'uncovering the knowledge implicit in practice means identifying knowledge that is generated by practitioners "solving" individual cases and problems and identifying how this contributes to the practitioner's personal store of experience' (Reed and Procter, 1993, p 163).

Many students experience role confusion, as they may have succeeded in other areas of their professional careers and find difficulty in accepting a colleague-teacher as more knowledgeable than they. Slavinsky and Diers (1982) found that post-registration students who are going through their own role conflict sometimes tend to be severe critics. Individuals will differ in previous achievements, knowledge and experience from their teachers, who may be more narrowly educated but, in a specialty area, be superior nurses.

Post-registration students may initially take a course for the primary reason of gaining an award and not for the value of the learning experience and the knowledge the award represents. They are likely to find the policies of the academic institution rigid, the cost, time and examinations frustrating and the course requirements a source of unnecessary obstacles to be overcome. Understanding this attitude is important in today's race for credentialism which puts pressures on registered nurses to 'keep up'. Time spent by teachers in the initial weeks of a course in explaining to students the nature of the course and the reasons for academic requirements is vital. Within a supporting relationship, frustrated students can receive support and assistance.

Needs as practitioners

The demands of post-registration students on teachers for teaching and supervising, especially as beginning learners in a new professional field, are great. Firstly, mature students are often ashamed to ask for extra help and support, preferring to 'tough it out'. Understandably, disclosing the need for assistance in nursing practice from one nurse professional to another could be seen as demeaning.

Hengstberger-Sims (1987) found that, depending on the number of years since active professional work, registered nurses' knowledge of current theory, drugs and side effects, professional skills and practices was understandably inadequate. They were not confident in their own skills nor were they capable of taking responsibility for patient care without supervision.

Many students returning to practice after an absence of some years have been strongly influenced in the past by the medical model. Their expectations of clinical practice with a familiar approach to patient care as they knew it will not be met. Sessions of briefing and debriefing, reflecting on practice, even nursing care plans will be new learning to many and may be seen as unnecessary and a waste of time.

Stoner, Collins and Yetton (1985) insist that it is essential that in working with new practitioners their teachers or supervisors have appropriate skills. Some post-registration students are threatening to teachers. 'It takes personal and professional maturity for faculty to work well with students who are by definition intelligent, inquisitive and aggressive' (Slavinsky and Diers, 1982).

TEACHING POST-REGISTRATION STUDENTS IN THE WORKPLACE

ACTIVITY

How can learning in the workplace be designed to meet the special needs of post-registration students? Refer to the principles of learning in the workplace and to the needs of post-registration students and identify the guidelines you would use to select learning strategies for this group of students.

FEEDBACK

Basing the selection of learning strategies on a set of criteria is useful as it helps to focus on learning that is relevant to learners' (rather than teachers') needs as well as to acknowledge that there are principles of learning in the workplace that can guide learning programmes.

A commonly used set of criteria governing workplace experience is:

- developing inquiry, critical thinking and critical reflectivity;
- developing self-direction, empowerment and political skills in learning and working;
- recognizing, contributing to and nurturing a supportive learning environment in the workplace;
- recognizing the complexity of the organizational context in which learning and working take place.

Each of these criteria is expanded below.

DEVELOPING INQUIRY, CRITICAL THINKING AND CRITICAL REFLECTIVITY

Below are some learning strategies which have been tried successfully in post-registration courses.

Developing inquiry skills

Problem-based learning

Higgins (1994) introduced the method into a class of post-registration students as a way of providing a strategy to meet the diverse needs and experiences of post-registration students.

A learning context was provided in which students drew on their clinical experience, practical and personal knowledge and their knowledge from the academic course. Working in groups students shared their perceptions of a 'real-life' problem and discussed possible interventions. Each stage was accompanied by challenges to each student's interpretations and conclusions. In addition, 'the flexible and student managed nature of PBL could help to accommodate individual differences and could give considerable scope for interactive and collaborative learning' (Higgins, 1994, p 25).

Action learning

This method implies the need to take action in the workplace; to be active rather than passive. Essentially it is a form of learning by experience through solving a real problem (Marsick, 1991). MacNamara, Meyler and Arnold (1990) trace the concept of action learning to the work of Revans (1980) and claim that it is a term for a model of problem-solving and self-development that emphasizes learning by doing. Marsick (1987) clarifies this position by pointing to the essential difference between problem-solving and action learning, describing the latter as 'a form of inquiry that combines investigation with action'. The necessity to follow through and actually implement change in the workplace draws on critical reflection and empowers the participants as they work in groups and reflect on their assumptions, values and actions. Action-learning programmes provide a framework for learning from experience 'involving reflection, that typically involves critical reflection, and that can – when well designed – involve critical self-reflection' (Marsick, 1991, p 25).

Working in groups on a real problem in the workplace is particularly appropriate for management courses for post-registration students. Assuming that the participants are employed in the same institution or community facility, an 'action learning set' of four or five students, including an adviser, is formed. The group serves as a resource and provides members with emotional support during discussion and critical reflection at each stage of the action.

While it can be introduced as the application of academic principles to practice, action learning can be a successful method of examining clinical practice and developing principles from practice. Action learning can be a way of learning research methods, of learning organizational skills and of practising communication and interviewing skills. To the extent that students can learn to effect change by action research, they learn the value of critical reflection on each step of achieving results. Reflections on self-image as a change agent, and weighing up the effects of personal behaviour on others in the workplace, leads to developing skills of critical reflectivity appropriate to the workplace.

Developing critical thinking skills

Developing critical thinking skills is vital in post-registration students.

Brookfield (1991, p 20–21) gives three reasons for the development of critical thinking skills: it is one of the intellectual functions most characteristic of adult life, it is necessary for personal survival and it is politically necessary in a democratic society. In an earlier discussion, Brookfield (1989, p 7–8) identifies the components of critical thinking:

- challenging assumptions;
- challenging the importance of context;
- imagining and exploring alternatives.

'The central value of critical thinking lies in its emancipatory potential' (Kramer, 1993, p 407). 'Emancipatory learning' has been adapted from the work of Habermas (1979). Individuals are freed to see new directions and new possibilities in their own lives, their surroundings and their world. For post-registration learning in the workplace there is freedom in gaining increased understanding of personal relationships, in re-evaluating personal perspectives, in recognizing that tolerance for different views is increased as understanding different positions is realized. Political skills are increased as students learn to question and examine the basis of values and meanings.

Emancipatory teaching

How can learners be involved in developing critical thinking skills? Burrows (1993) proposes emancipatory teaching; critical thinking is promoted though dialogue.

Used as part of staff development, learning emancipatory skills in the workplace can empower RNs to begin lifelong development of critical thinking skills. 'Both teacher and learner participate in acquiring knowledge, reflecting on options and evaluating strategies' (p 33). The emancipated teacher–learner relationship is highly appropriate for staff development programmes. It provides encouragement for continually probing experiences, trying to discover why they are or are not effective and learning how to change if necessary.

Burrows cites three examples of emancipatory teaching: clinical judgement seminars, case studies or simulations and journal writing.

- **Clinical judgement seminars.** In this method a critical incident is presented by one of the student group. Through non-judgemental questioning the incident is thoroughly explored and 'the richness of clinical practice knowing can be uncovered' (Burrows, 1993, p 33). There are a few ground rules to ensure that the clinical judgement seminar is productive:
  - the source of the story should be identified;
  - the storyteller must take responsibility for her or his actions in the situation;
  - the stories and subsequent actions should be purposeful;
  - the listeners should understand the reasons why the teller is sharing the story;
  - the storyteller's feelings, ideas and experience should be related to the group;

- the storyteller must be cautious about using information that could hurt another person;
- the storyteller should point out opportunities for growth in self and others;
- humour can be used constructively to address feelings and explore aspects of a situation;
- storytelling must not be used to ridicule or diminish group members.

- **Simulations.** Group discussion and analysis of case studies or simulations focus students' attention on the process of solving the simulated problem rather than on the solution. Participation is increased by each group member assuming the role of discussion guide, learning the skills of guiding a group through emphasizing the need to keep an open mind, questioning, reflecting on information, reasoning and suspending judgement.

- **Journal writing.** Practising journal writing can be commenced within a post-registration course by writing a 10–15-minute journal entry before, during or after a workplace learning session. Writing about a critical incident in which their actions made a difference provides excellent material for developing reflective, analytical and creative expression (Burrows, 1993).

In general, journal-keeping is an effective way to enable students to reflect on their learning experiences in order to:
- keep track of their goals and how they are progressing toward them;
- review the strategies they use;
- analyse the way they learn;
- trace their development in becoming self-aware;
- review the log to inter-relate their ideas;
- record 'discoveries' in clinical practice.

Developing critical reflectivity

The capacity for critical self-reflection is a characteristic of professional practice. Linked with critical thinking in its challenge of workplace assumptions and practice routines, it goes further. According to Schon (1988), critical reflectivity is seen best in uncertain, unique and conflicting situations of practice where guidelines for action are unavailable. When a practitioner goes beyond accepted styles of thinking and practice to systematically examine what is being done and can be done, then to reflect on it, leading to action – this is what Schon (1988) calls 'reflection-in-action'.

Because of the different conditions in the workplace where reflective and critically reflective workplace learning occurs, Marsick (1987) believes that an exact recipe for workplace learning cannot be provided. Some strategies that encourage reflective activity and which through mentoring and coaching guide practitioners through the stages of critical reflectivity are:

- well remembered events;
- role play, role reversal and critical debates;
- support groups.

Well remembered events

Recording well remembered events resembles journal writing in that an event, an incident or an episode that a student observes in a particular situation and considers for his or her own reasons especially salient or memorable are recorded. Critical phases and critical persons as well as critical incidents can be the focus for recording well remembered events. Critical thinking is a process, not an outcome (Brookfield, 1989) so the events are recorded over a period and changes in behaviour, practices or approaches can be subject to reflective analysis. The analysis can be personal or shared in a group. 'In comparing vividly remembered episodes, insulting or affirming actions or methods that worked especially well, (practitioners) gain insights into which features of their practice hold true across settings and which are specific to a certain context' (Brookfield, 1989, p 41). The relevance to workplace learning in a nursing environment is obvious. Well remembered events are described at weekly intervals. As new or returning graduates record their interpretation of events, over time, it is possible for them to gain insights into what they know and how their knowledge changes.

Role play

Role play is described in Chapter 4. Our intention here is to emphasize the value of role play in fostering critical reflectivity by learning to examine taken-for-granted assumptions in the workplace and challenging values that can often undermine practice. Learning about one's workplace practice brings workplace reality into the role play. This can bring out the difference between knowing what to do and doing it (Marsick, 1987).

Support networks

Nurses supporting nurses in 'a good new nurse network' 'could be a source of encouragement for the nurse who takes risks in her professional setting . . . a strong nursing network could encourage peer relationships and peer groups that could share information, review work and provide feedback, explore issues and strategies, and assist each other in problem-solving techniques' (Hamilton, 1981, p 4). Smythe (1984) also claims that social support groups in the workplace provide emotional support, offer protection against stress and, through the support of an expert nurse, can provide valuable corrective feedback of nursing practice.

DEVELOPING SELF-DIRECTION, EMPOWERMENT AND POLITICAL SKILLS

Self-directed learning

Self-directed learning describes a process in which individuals take the initiative, with or without the help of others, in diagnosing their learning needs, formulating learning goals, identifying human and material resources for learning, choosing and implementing appropriate learning strategies and evaluating learning outcomes (Knowles, 1975, p 18). Although the concept has been researched extensively over the last decade there is still no widely accepted alternative to Knowles's early definition. Self-directed learning and independent learning are discussed at length in Chapter 4. Our focus in this chapter is on self-directed learning by RNs new to learning in the workplace and as professionals developing skills in returning to learning.

Reflection-in-action

Reflection-in-action is at the heart of self-directed learning in the workplace.

This implies that teachers and learners are involved in a process of inquiry and analysis: teachers to support and encourage, learners to recognize and diagnose their learning needs. The capacity of the work environment to support self-directed learning implies that an active learning environment exists with recognition of the importance of individual learners.

Examples of the learning needs some RNs could choose for self-directed learning are:

- communication skills with patients or clients, with other professionals, administrators and non-professional staff;
- caring for challenging patients or clients;
- conducting patient or client teaching;
- being aware of own reactions and emotions;

- progress in technical skills;
- turning negative experience into learning;
- tracing self-growth over an agreed period.

Learning to learn in the workplace needs teachers with facilitation skills who will encourage learners to recognize the informal learning occurring as they examine what happened in clinical practice. This leads to increased self-direction in learning as 'learning awareness' is sharpened.

Learning contracts

A learning contract can be thought of as a way of structuring self-directed learning. A major difference is that the format of the contract allows for assessment. In clinical practice this could be an important strategy for increasing learners' self-awareness in judging how they are improving. Setting targets in the form of clinical or personal objectives to be met as well as the criteria by which the performance is to be judged is accepting a learning and performance challenge that can have lifelong learning benefits. The rewards are in terms of increased self-confidence in managing learning experiences.

A typical learning contract contains four categories: objectives, resources, implementation and evaluation.

- **Objectives.** The teacher's facilitation skills are required at each stage of the contract being formulated. In framing objectives, the learner needs to consider whether the objectives are realistic, appropriate for the time available and important enough for the stage of learning. Framing an objective such as 'on fulfilment of this contract the student will be more able to uncover the hidden knowledge in clinical practice', the learner may need guidance in identifying what exactly is meant, and then reframing the overall objective into smaller stepwise objectives. Preferably the objective should also include ways the objective will be met, e.g. 'to reflect on the meaning of an episode of clinical practice by discussing what happened with the facilitator'.
- **Resources.** Identifying resources involves the learner in, for example, selection of literature, naming resource persons, patients and clients, selecting appropriate time and clinical environment.
- **Implementation.** Arrange briefing and debriefing sessions with the facilitator. Draw on models of debriefing to record observations, discussions, discoveries and future decisions about own learning in clinical practice.

- **Evaluation.** Post-registration students in the workplace can write the criteria for their reflective practice. Obviously this will differ according to the individual and the workplace.

Empowerment

Mentoring

As a way of learning through relationships with other people, mentoring has many different descriptions in nursing literature. In this chapter we will refer to mentoring as a supportive guide at critical stages in post-registration learning. This could be during transition to a new environment or to a change or role in the same institution. The closeness of the two-way relationship is its most outstanding feature. Jowers and Herr (1990) provide an example of a mentor, the leader in a primary team nursing approach who gave direct patient care and provided a role model for the team. In another example the mentor and a clinical nurse worked on patient-care assignments with the mentor providing support and intervention in ongoing nursing care when appropriate. Certainly there are similarities between mentoring and preceptoring, with added roles for the mentor in providing career advice and grooming practitioners for future professional advancement.

In Jowers and Herr's report (1990), the dilemmas and barriers of mentor relationships are listed. Potential problems include: overprotection by the mentor; potential for exploitation; confusion between educator and mentor roles; possibility of protégés becoming clones of the mentor rather than autonomous individuals.

Job assignments

Learning through job assignments promotes breadth, leadership, visibility and responsibility. During re-entry courses or clinical specialization courses the attachment of the student to a special area with a preceptor, mentor or coach allows the student to accept job challenges and difficulties, for example, making mistakes and accepting correction (McCauley, 1986).

Political skills

Most teachers and learners would admit that learning is change. As complex as the process of change is, again, most teachers and learners would consider with Brookfield (1991) that there are always political dimensions to change. 'For teachers and students, nothing is exactly the same after an educational event as it was before' (p 187). The important question is, in what direction is change occurring during the process of our teaching and learning? What values are operative in the way learning is planned, learners are encouraged and evaluation of performance is conducted?

When RNs return to practice after an extended period of absence they may expect the same conditions to operate as when they were students. The skills that current students acquire in asking awkward questions about why circumstances are as they appear, whose interests are being served and how things could be changed may not have been learned in the past and may also be regarded as not quite 'proper' in a professional person. They may be surprised to find included in their course, and as essentials in workplace learning, skills to challenge the accuracy and validity of some of the 'givens' around them and to practise being 'thinkingly active'. Some of the popular teaching in assertiveness training has addressed these issues. What we are emphasizing here is that present-day health professionals, and particularly nurses, need to develop skills of political reasoning.

What does this mean for workplace learning and teaching? Most nurses would agree that political survival in an institution is learned on the job. Power plays and shifting priorities often determine how effective practitioners can be in giving a caring service to patients and clients. New staff returning to practice or moving to a new institution need to discover the communication channels and the centres of power and influence in the new environment.

What can the teacher do to assist? It is important to approach discussion of the political culture of the organization through some of the accepted learning strategies. Talking about the political culture of an organization can be dealt with through:

- critical incident exercises;
- debating.

Critical incident exercise

Participants in groups of four are asked to think back to a time when they felt threatened by political developments in their institution (examples could be closure of hospital wards, cessation of a community health project or closure of a whole hospital). Each participant records the event, who was involved, how they responded to the event and the consequence of the event for them personally and professionally. The group then comes together, compares and collates individual accounts, identifying similarities in the nature of the threats faced and the responses made. As a result of the exercise some basic notes about political survival emerge. These can be recorded, together with common mistakes, political errors and other comments. To take the exercise further, participants at a later date could apply what they have learned to an imminent event in their own practical situation.

Debating

This method provides opportunities for investigating and analysing issues thoroughly, for presenting ideas clearly and for recognizing flaws in arguments. Debates start with a solution – unlike discussion or problem-solving, where the conclusion is unknown. The learning for the student is in seeing how:

> the choice of a particular viewpoint or theoretical framework influences the selection, analysis, and interpretation of supporting data. The theoretical framework governs not only the selection of facts to be used in the argument, but also the analysis and interpretation of those facts. With the explicit shift in a debate format, students are better able to critically examine the basis of their stands on issues.
>
> *(Source: Gesse and Dempsey, 1981, p 424)*

How can debates be used in workplace learning? Choose an organizational topic for debate; or focus on an imminent clinical change to debate the pros and cons. Critical debate is a particular kind of role reversal where participants are asked 'to explore an idea or take a position that they find unsympathetic, immoral or distasteful' (Brookfield, 1991, p 129).

CREATING A SUPPORTIVE LEARNING ENVIRONMENT IN THE WORKPLACE

ACTIVITY

Any location in the workplace needs to be recognized for its potential as a learning as well as working environment. Check the characteristics of a learning environment (Marsick, 1987) earlier in this chapter. Are there any you could add after considering the workplace teaching you are involved in with post-registration students? What learning strategies could you introduce so that students learn to nurture a learning environment?

FEEDBACK

The working and learning environment of nursing can be stressful. Another characteristic to be added is that a positive learning environment recognizes potential stressors and introduces supportive measures. An effective supportive learning environment 'must provide opportunities for experimentation, risk-taking, dialogue, initiative, creativity and participation in decision-making' (Marsick, 1987, p 25).

Experiencing a positive learning environment contributes to 'work excitement', where learners share their experiences with others who, in turn, incorporate innovations into their practice. Lickman, Simms and Greene (1993) report that a learning environment which fosters individual growth and development provides a variety of experiences and positive working conditions. Descriptions of a workplace as energized and exhilarated may be associated with 'high-tech' acute care. However, Baldwin and Price (1994) found that 'nurses with higher levels of work excitement selected home care because of personal fulfilment, whereas those who were less excited chose home care for schedule flexibility'. A positive learning environment depends not so much on the perception of 'high-' or 'low-tech' but on how the participants energize themselves and each other in developing learning communities.

Teachers can point to opportunistic learning in the workplace that students could overlook.

- Accompany students in 'hands-on' activities and ask them what they observe every day that could present 'hidden' knowledge if investigated. Share the suggestions later with the group.
- Encourage learners to jot down brief notes on different or surprising opportunities to be shared in the total group later.
- Involve students in suggesting a small clinical practice study based on their diagnosis of a clinical problem.
- Invite students to design a learning package for the next group of post-registration students entering the workplace.

In summary, the energy generated by involvement, positive feedback and support, injects the learning community with a new and heightened awareness of the possibilities of workplace learning.

RECOGNIZING THE COMPLEXITY OF THE ORGANIZATIONAL CONTEXT OF THE WORKING AND LEARNING ENVIRONMENT

Learning how to manage the work environment is a hurdle for post-registration students. What learning strategies can be used in the workplace?

- Understanding structures.
- Understanding how value structure, informal and formal goal structure, norms, roles, power and authority hierarchies influence the workplace can be mysterious to RNs new to the workplace. Learning strategies whereby written organizational charts are compared with how the workplace actually functions can be discussed in workplace groups. Examples of situations where values of the workplace are in contrast to individual values can be the focus of discussion or role plays.
- **Communicating in the workplace.** Words used in the context of patient care can often be dehumanizing. Invite the students to make lists of words or phrases heard in the workplace and in a group context focus the discussion on the opposites. For example, the lists could be 'humanizing/dehumanizing' words, 'personal/impersonal' or 'technical/expressive'.

Tracing the communication patterns in the unit is a valuable learning exercise. Who talks to whom? For how long and how frequently? Among a group of patients the culture and language differences may result in some patients being isolated.

Following a written communication through the organizational structure can be instructive about facilitative or obstructive communication.

A final comment from Marsick (1987) captures the importance of consideration of the workers and learners as individuals in any organization.

Current training models emphasize job-related knowledge and skills as if it is possible to divorce them from the rest of the worker's life. However, for learning to be effective, one must consider at least two deeper levels in which job skills are embedded: the social unit that shapes the individual's actions at work, that is the organization and the immediate work group and the individual's perception of self *vis-à-vis* the job and the organization. Thus learning for organizational productivity cannot be divorced from learning for personal growth as is often done, nor can the burden of change be placed primarily on the individual in isolation from the organization.

(Source: Marsick, 1987, p 16)

SUMMARY

In summary, this chapter has identified some of the important issues of workplace teaching and learning. The topic took a wide sweep to include new graduates entering the professional nursing field, as well as postgraduate students returning to study and registered nurses returning to the workforce after an absence of some years. Several issues in the needs of registered nurses as learners, professionals and practitioners raised important considerations for workplace teachers in designing and implementing learning programmes that consider the person as well as the job.

Many issues remain unresolved, others were merely touched on. Hopefully, the literature resources and your experiences of workplace teaching will enable you and your colleagues, through critical reflection, to arrive at insights into the richness of day-to-day teaching and learning in the workplace.

Learning about values, human rights and ethics

7

INTRODUCTION

In the decade since this chapter was first written advances in technology have given society access to treatments in health care previously undreamed of, and at the same time have added considerably to the ethical considerations for nurses and nurse education. The ethical issues contained in genetic therapy, organ donation and the access of postmenopausal women to childbirth have claimed wide media attention. In addition, conditions such as HIV/AIDS have focused clearly on issues of discrimination and on the equitable distribution of expensive resources for care and research. Interventions such as the much publicized use of Dr Kervorkian's 'medicide' machine by some of his patients has sharpened the issues of euthanasia and brought the debate into the community graphically through television as well as print media. There should be no surprise, therefore, that the increasing concern for informed debate is reflected in the nursing literature. The study of nursing ethics is increasingly a part of both undergraduate and postgraduate curricula in nursing (Thompson, Melia and Boyd, 1988; Hunt, 1992; Johnstone, 1994).

We have selected values, ethical dilemmas and human rights for attention in this chapter as these aspects of contemporary nursing are gaining in importance as ethical problems increase. Teachers themselves are sometimes faced with ethical dilemmas in teaching and in nursing practice. They must also give support to students and colleagues who may be seeking to resolve an ethical dilemma. Obviously, the issues raised in teaching a component of values, human rights and ethics in a nursing curriculum are far more extensive than can be addressed in one chapter. Each requires a chapter in its own right, and even then the subject would not be fully addressed, so wide are the issues for health care and for education.

By the end of this chapter you should have examined some of the issues in teaching ethics and you should be able to design and manage learning sessions for students to increase their skills in:

- clarifying values;
- analysing human rights;
- resolving ethical dilemmas.

While the methods described in the previous chapters are appropriate for teaching most subjects and are appropriate in most situations, some adaptations are suggested in this chapter. The alternatives are offered to complement your usual teaching methods and to add to your repertoire of teaching skills. It is for you to decide whether they are appropriate for your purposes in assisting students in your particular programme.

CURRICULUM ISSUES

The curriculum issue is in capturing sufficient curriculum time to allow undergraduate and postgraduate students to reflect on their observations and reactions and to discuss the ethical conflicts they experience in practice. Kermode and Brown (1995) raise doubts about the existence of sufficient will and skill among nurses to engage in critiques of themselves and their occupation. If that is so, including 'critical ethics' in the curriculum should no longer be questioned.

At the outset it should be said that, to be most effective, teaching about values, human rights, moral reasoning and ethical decision-making should be an integral part of the curriculum. This is not to say that a large proportion of curriculum time should be devoted to these areas, but rather to make the point that adding on to an established curriculum is less than satisfactory and leads to teaching that is fragmented and often not in tune with the philosophical base of the programme. On the other hand, a curriculum that has been designed from concepts such as the nature of humankind or human needs would have identified the salient issues of values and human rights, and would have included the need for ethical decision-making as a required skill.

Your situation may not be able to accommodate a full course on nursing ethics within the curriculum and you may be faced with a decision to include or not to include ethics at all. In spite of the obvious pitfalls of a short course, many teachers would prefer to design a few brief sessions as a sensitization to the issues in nursing ethics rather than not including the subject, because of the need to include this important dimension in nursing practice and education.

Although nursing ethics is now a subject for study in its own right (Johnstone, 1994; Thompson, Melia and Boyd, 1988) and a considerable body of knowledge exists, in this text we are dealing with a process – a way of thinking – and the personal development that accompanies it, rather than a substantive content area to be explained. The process of becoming a nurse is achieved through a very efficient socialization process. The learning issue arises from the students' need to come to terms with conflicting values in the practice of nursing, particularly in the early years. As Thompson, Melia and Boyd (1988) point out, there is often tension for individual nurses in adopting professional values when they conflict with their own personal values.

It is, of course, not surprising that the hidden curriculum in the form of the socialization process makes students want to know how to master skills, behaviours and attitudes which will bring rewards of approval and acceptance within a hierarchical professional system. Nevertheless, the students' questions are often ethical questions that arise during everyday clinical practice.

Lutz, Elfrink and Eddy (1991), in their review of research on values and values education in nursing, point to the tendency of nurse educators to include values not in the formal programme but in incidental teaching as the need arises. The contrast with the teaching of scientific knowledge and psychomotor skills is obvious. One could argue that the place of values education is during clinical practice as practitioners confront values conflicts as a daily occurrence. However, Lutz, Elfrink and Eddy (1991) point out that, because values education has had such a minor role in the curriculum, practising nurses 'may not have the necessary knowledge and skills needed to fulfil their emerging practice role as autonomous moral decision-makers' (p 130).

TEACHING AND LEARNING ISSUES

Deciding what to teach (Chapter 2) and arranging the conditions most likely to bring about learning (Chapter 3) have their foundation in accepted educational principles; so also does the design of teaching sessions (Chapter 4). Yet, in spite of the expertise a teacher may possess in modifying educational principles for a particular learning situation, and the enthusiasm brought to the teaching of a subject, students often respond more to the pressures for socialization into the mores of hospital practice than to lifelong learning skills of gaining knowledge and applying it to practice.

The important links between what is being taught and the student's personal growth are tenuous, if ever made explicit, and the rewards for students are virtually non-existent. Most students want to know more than what to do, or what to know – they are 'whole' people too and they search for meaning. What does this mean for me? How ought I to behave? What is the 'right' action for me in this or that situation?

For individual students, the search for meaning is personal: it holds the key to personal growth and has the potential for lifting ideas out of the everyday commonplace to increasing levels of understanding of themselves and others. Personal knowledge is at the heart of values clarification, which in turn influences decisions taken in patient interaction. Kasch (1986) declares that 'competent nursing action is likely to be a function of the nurse's understanding of self and other, i.e., the level of person knowledge'. It is this dimension that is so important to capture in teaching values, human rights and ethics. The rigidity and blandness suggested by formal codes of ethics should in no way prejudice us about the nature of thinking about ethical issues.

On the other hand, the pressures on teachers to teach a packed course and to cover the content sometimes results in the hasty selection of teaching materials and experiences. Teachers new to an area such as nursing ethics may find that their trusted skills in other content areas of the curriculum are not as appropriate and different teaching approaches are needed. 'The educators need to be re-educated' (Hunt, 1992).

How then should teaching strategies be selected? The usual answer is to consult the aims and learning objectives of the subject in which the expected outcomes will be defined. On the other hand, your programme may have teaching objectives but not learning objectives, and you will need to convert them (see Chapter 3).

Lutz, Elfrink and Eddy (1991) provide suggestions about what could be done to stimulate strategies for engaging students in learning opportunities. The use of frameworks through which students learn an approach to values, ethical and moral conflicts and human rights issues appears to offer the most effective foundation for classroom discussion, which can then be followed through into clinical practice. It follows that nurse educators need to be better prepared to design curricula which include a component of values teaching/learning and also be better equipped to design learning strategies.

Lamenting on the limited teaching/learning strategies they discovered in schools of nursing in the USA, Lutz, Elfrink and Eddy (1991) point to the importance of including values so that students would learn to examine value conflicts, 'which are the foundation to understanding ethical and moral dilemmas' (p 135).

ISSUES OF NURSING PRACTICE

An interesting debate in nursing centres on an analysis of care and whether there can be an ethics of care (Allmark, 1995). Humanizing health care continues to be a priority for nurses just as it is for most health workers. Technology and technological change have the power to both elevate and degrade the care that nurses give. Teachers of nurses are therefore in a position of paramount importance in assisting students to work their way through the ethical, moral and value conflicts that will confront them from time to time.

'The task confronting nursing at this time is not to articulate its philosophy of care better than it has already done, not to define precisely the concept of care itself (this may not be possible), but to make **care** (as it has been articulated to date) more visible as something to be valued both as a virtue and as a principle' (Johnstone, 1994, p 133). In this respect Johnstone claims that nursing needs to be better informed about 'the development of a substantive moral theory' to which nursing has a contribution to make.

Assisting students to understand the ethic of care, which is recognized as the imperative of nursing and, indeed, its moral foundation, is a task for clinical practitioners as well as educators. To engage in reflective thinking about what has been observed is a dimension of ethical analysis.

SUMMARY

In summary, then, to be effective, a course in nursing ethics (including values and human rights), preferably:

- is integrated within the curriculum;
- is designed to facilitate the personal growth of students;
- provides time and guidance for reflective and critical thinking;
- produces skills to use in the resolution of ethical dilemmas of real people.

VALUES

ACTIVITY

While it is true that values are involved in all we do and influence the decisions and choices we make, the concept of value is not easy to define. What do you mean by value(s)?

FEEDBACK

There are similarities in the definitions of values in the writings of contemporary and earlier researchers. For Raths (1966, p 38) values are 'guides to behaviour that evolve and mature, . . . are seen as worthy, and give direction to life'. Hill (1991, p 4) claims that 'when people speak of "values" they are usually referring to those beliefs held by individuals to which they attach special priority or worth, and by which they tend to order their lives'. You will find slight variations in Reilly (1989) and Lemin, Potts and Welsford (1994), among many others, yet, interestingly, they complement one another. Particularly for nursing, the 'guides to action' are significant. 'A link can be made between the action-orientation of values (. . .) and the role of values in mediating the decision making of nurses' (Lutz, Elfrink and Eddy, 1991).

Hill (1991) claims that a value is more than a belief and also more than a feeling. It has three elements: a cognitive element, the belief statement being referred to as a 'value judgement'; an affective element, often spoken of as 'attitudes'; and a volitional element that influences the choices we make so that they are consistent with the beliefs and values.

VALUES EDUCATION

ACTIVITY

You have offered to take responsibility for the introduction of a series of sessions on nursing ethics for students in a basic programme. The course has three components: values, human rights and ethics. You are preparing to teach the values component. What do you hope your students will derive from it?

FEEDBACK

You may be teaching in a programme where ethics (including values and human rights) is a separate course or an elective subject. In that case you will be able to plan a course so that time is available for students to reflect on some of the issues in value development and values clarification. Your expectation would be that the students would gain an understanding of the values they hold. This would serve as a preparation for ethical decision-making later as they take more responsibility in the care of patients. On the other hand your programme may not devote so much time to ethics but may acknowledge the importance of values by allotting special sessions during an intensive-care or coronary-care course.

There are alternative arrangements for including values clarification in the programme although a whole session may not be given over to the topic. For example, in clinical practice or community placements, the pre- and post-clinical conference can offer a special opportunity for choosing and clarifying values. For example, the knowledge necessary for nursing a patient with multiple fractures and internal injuries following a car accident could be followed by revision of the skills of observation, technical treatment, basic care and planning a rehabilitation programme. Lastly, the fact that the patient has been charged with drunken driving in an accident which killed a child calls into question the effectiveness of nursing the patient if the values dimension has not been faced openly and explored.

Values education can also be built into subject matter. 'Values education is reflected in the choice of topic, people and events studied, the resources used, and the methods of teaching and learning employed' (Lemin, Potts and Welsford, 1994). Perhaps this is obvious to most teachers but it is fairly common in practice to find that teachers may exhibit their own values on a particular issue (for example, the right to life movement) but omit values clarification as a means of opening up or expanding students' skill in recognizing their own values. Needless to say, the important point is that at some time during the course students need to learn the process of valuing.

In summary your learning objectives for students in the values component of the course in nursing ethics would be, broadly:

- gaining an understanding of our own personal values;
- using the process of valuing;
- recognizing personal and professional values.

VALUES CLARIFICATION AND VALUES INQUIRY

A useful distinction between values clarification and values inquiry is made by Schoenly (1994). Identification of personal beliefs and values and sharing these with others describes values clarification; values inquiry centres on values in social and moral issues. Schoenly cites the investigation of incidents in newspaper accounts which are value-laden as an example of values inquiry. In a cultural diversity programme, understanding different nursing situations may require inquiry into the value systems of a variety of ethnic and cultural groups.

VALUES CLARIFICATION

ACTIVITY

You have decided to introduce first-year students to values clarification. As this will be a departure from their usual format of lectures and group discussion on the substantive content of the course, how will you prepare the students for your session?

FEEDBACK

You could apply the principles of 'advance organizers' discussed in Chapter 3. This would help students to prepare for learning about values by linking it to their past learning or experiences.

For example, questions might be related to a recent class, such as: 'During the lecture in paediatric nursing several students took issue with the case history presented of child abuse. What was your view? Why?'

Ask five friends, colleagues or family members to complete a sentence or two, such as: 'Euthanasia in this country is . . . '. 'What I value most in life is . . . '. (The topic of the sentence should be chosen to provide the link with a previous session.) Bring the completed statements to the values class.

As well as acting as advance organizers, the answers students bring to class provide a warming-up period at the beginning of the session. It is often useful to have a poster wall of issues to work from. Students' contributions written or drawn on butcher's paper can be displayed anonymously at first, then acknowledged later when the group is felt to be supportive for its members.

ACTIVITY

As a facilitator in the values-clarification session you will have chosen an informal setting and arranged a comfortable atmosphere and encouraged the display of posters around the room. What will you do next?

FEEDBACK

The first time you conduct a values-exploration session you will probably over-prepare for it. That is an advantage as you can use whichever strategy appears to be appropriate to the group's progress. The methods you choose depend on how well you know the group and also on your perception of the importance of the development and clarification of values.

First, it is important for you to explain to the students the purpose and the ground rules of the session: 'You will learn ways of valuing – not a particular set of values; it is for you to discover where you stand on issues you may be facing; you are allowed to have "time out" on an issue if you don't wish to discuss your particular stance'.

Second, you may also consider it is important to spend a short few minutes confiding your understanding of the process of valuing to the group. For instance, you may wish the group to be aware that you recognize in teachers, parents and authorities several forms of valuing, for example:

- **moralizing** – pressing on others one's view of what is right or wrong;
- *laissez-faire* – leaving values up to chance;
- **modelling** – trying to make practice and ideals match;
- **values identification and clarification** – building one's own values system (Simon, Howe and Kerschenbaum, 1978).

The group's reaction would be very interesting at this point and could be elicited by asking students to write a slogan to fit each of the four types, then discussing the comparative forms of valuing. For example:

Value form	Slogan
Moralizing	People who don't care don't deserve care
Laissez-faire	Who cares?
Modelling	I care, between 9 am and 5 pm
Values clarification	Caring costs; but I choose to care

Third, with the group relaxed and the butcher's-paper wall posters as a backdrop, one of the 'strategies frameworks' of values clarification would be introduced, preferably as a brief handout with discussion. The purpose would be to use the framework for guidance in clarifying the values brought to class.

An early framework is Raths's 'theory of valuing' (Raths, 1966). The human being can arrive at values by an intelligent process of choosing, prizing and behaving.

- **Choosing:**
1. freely;
2. from alternatives;
3. after thoughtful consideration of the consequences of each alternative.
- **Prizing:**
4. cherishing, being happy with the choice;
5. willing to affirm the choice publicly.
- **Acting:**
6. doing something with the choice;
7. repeatedly, in some pattern of life.

(Source: adapted from Simon, Howe and Kerschenbaum, 1978. An abbreviated form of this framework in the form of a schematic outline of the criteria for values is given by Lutz, Elfrink and Eddy, 1991, p 132)

Fourth, returning to the wall posters, group members could explain the value they had identified, obtain clarification and consider the consequences of an alternative choice (Steps 1, 2 and 3, above) to test the strength of the value (Step 4, above). A useful strategy is to involve the whole group in forming a continuum. This is done by individuals taking a position on an imaginary line from positive at one end of the line to negative at the opposite end. The students place themselves at appropriate points on the continuum to express the strength of their view. This often results in clarification as rethinking and repositioning occurs following hearing from other students the justification they have given for their position. The aim is to enable students to obtain feedback on their statement of the values they purport to hold. This strategy is also a dramatic way of demonstrating that issues are rarely clear-cut with a unanimous black or white decision.

Fifth, being comfortable with the choice of a value leads to a willingness to affirm it publicly (Step 5, above). In class this can be done by sending an imaginary facsimile message – an 'I urge you' fax. Blank fax forms can be supplied to add a touch of realism, and the strategy works best if the subject of the fax is a topical issue and the recipient is sufficiently prominent to excite imaginative messages. For example, an 'I urge you' fax to the Minister for Health following the decision to close city hospitals or reduce a community health programme could generate a number of values.

- I urge you to close hospital X, not my hospital.
- I urge you to close more beds: this country is over-supplied.
- I urge you to think of students who need sufficient clinical material on which to learn.

The fax should be made public; the sender should give the justification, aided by the group, who should question and comment until the value is affirmed or denied.

Sixth, this would be an appropriate point to clarify with the group what congruence they can identify between their personal values and the professional values they have observed so far in their experience. Depending on the level of your group you could proceed by:

- setting group tasks based on the students' suggestions of points for clarification;
- setting group tasks by assigning to each a clause from the international code of nursing ethics and comparing the values expressed in it with the personal values affirmed earlier by the group.

As a summary, a plan of possible strategies is given in Table 7.1. The size of your student group, the time and the resources available together with your personal preferences and the level of your group will determine which of the strategies you wish to use or adapt.

Table 7.1   Summary of suggested plan for values-clarification sessions

Objective	Teacher activity	Student activity
	Prepares group by giving advance organizers Arranges room Sets tone	Obtains data Records on wall posters
Uses the process of valuing	Give ground rules Gives own examples of valuing Introduces the Raths theory in stages Steps 1, 2 and 3	Discusses ground rules Writes slogans and discusses values Discusses theory Applies Steps 1, 2 and 3 of theory to values chosen from those recorded on wall posters
Gains an understanding of personal values	Step 4	Affirms and clarifies a value publicly
	Step 5	Acts on the value by an 'I urge you' fax
Recognizes personal professional values	Step 6	Compares personal and professional values
	Sets up group task and facilitates group interaction Summarizes Foreshadows work on human rights Makes links Closes session	

A criticism of values-clarification strategies is that the activity is an end in itself and fails to carry over into the students' learning. For some students this criticism would apply. According to Simon, Howe and Kerschenbaum (1978, p 20), there is empirical evidence that students who have taken part in values clarification have become less apathetic, less flighty, less conforming as well as less over-dissenting. They are more zestful and energetic, more critical in their thinking and are more likely to follow through on decisions.

Another criticism is that the act of choosing a value allows the individual to accept or reject certain values. Purtilo (1983) points out that, in nursing and the health professions generally, there are some values that logically follow if a concept such as 'treating the whole patient' is accepted. The reasoning is that the 'whole' person is not only a physical, emotional or spiritual being but also a moral being. Values such as quality of life, right of choice and self-determination are part of a professional ethic which, it is assumed, members of the profession not only accept but practise. Raths's (1966) theory of valuing is composed of seven processes, the last two being concerned with acting on one's belief. The assumption here is that the person will indicate what action will result from possessing and affirming a particular value.

Bernal and Bush (1985) offer criticism of values clarification as an inadequate form of resolving an ethical dilemma. We would agree, but we are not advocating values clarification as anything more than a way of enabling nurses to become aware of, and to identify more clearly, their personal values and to examine the conflicts between their personal and professional values.

VALUES INQUIRY

Transcultural nursing provides the nursing profession with one of its most powerful challenges. D'Cruz and Tham (1993) studied cultural, curriculum and demographic issues in one Australian state (Victoria). Their results showed that 43.6% of the population were born overseas or were Australian-born with one or both parents born overseas. The different interpretations of health and illness in such a multicultural society suggest that values inquiry skills are a necessary and important component of a nursing course.

Lemin, Potts and Welsford (1994) provide a 'values exploration' strategy in which they show how beliefs determine values, which underlie attitudes and are reflected in actions (p 4). The underlying convictions of Jewish/Christian, Koori (Australian Aboriginal), Buddhist and Islamic beliefs are briefly summarized; the 'standards of worth' and the underlying attitudes are followed by the actions (the ways we live out our attitudes) typical of each group. For example, the 'standards of worth' of Jewish/Christian groups is given as 'all beings are significant', the resulting attitude is 'you must care for others' and the actions are 'acts of love and kindness'. For the Koori group, 'the land and people are one' is given as the standard of worth, the underlying attitude is that 'you must care for the land' and the resulting action is 'caring and sharing – no ownership'.

For students of nursing the different reactions of indigenous and other cultural or religious groups to the values of the dominant society can be seen to have strong ideological and religious foundations. Using a values inquiry approach students can be helped to understand the health and illness behaviour of people from a variety of different cultural backgrounds.

HUMAN RIGHTS

We have now reached the point where we move from designing learning strategies for clarifying personal or individual values to those for teaching about shared values, or universal rights. However, there is merit in designing your sessions on human rights so that a direct link is made with the work your students have done on their own values. The reason is that students find the study of human rights (important though it is) to be remote if it drifts too soon into abstract statements and official declarations. After all, the aim of humanizing relationships in health care becomes meaningless to students if the method of teaching about human rights is so formal that it is routine, dull and boring – in a word, dehumanizing.

'What we have to respect are real people, not abstractions or sentimental idealizations' (Kamenka and Tay, 1981). Certainly, real people are affected, as Weeramantry (1981) notes:

Almost every advance of technology – nuclear, biological, medical, cybernetic – is fraught with limitless possibilities for the negation of human rights. The right to health and to a pure, unpolluted environment is imperilled by nuclear technology; the integrity of the human body by organ transplants, ectogenetic conception, *in vitro* fertilization, prenatal selection of sex and attributes; the integrity of the mind by psychosurgery and numerous techniques of mind manipulation; the baselines of freedom by cybernetic regulation; the essentials of privacy by dozens of surveillance devices ranging from bugging devices to long-distance scanners.

(Source: Weeramantry, 1981, p 50)

ACTIVITY

What are the learning objectives you consider are important for students to achieve by the end of the session(s) on human rights?

FEEDBACK

We should try to be as clear as possible about the learning objectives for students in these sessions. Again, we are assisting them in learning skills and in shaping attitudes.

Not a little confusion may be generated by the terms 'teaching human rights' or 'teaching about human rights', as if there exists somewhere a body of knowledge called 'human rights'.

Human rights in themselves are not matters of knowledge in the way that chemistry or biology are matters of knowledge. There can, of course, be knowledge about the laws that exist to protect human rights and there can be knowledge about the history or sociology of human rights, but the existence of human rights themselves is a matter of opinion and questions about specific human rights are also matters of opinion (Singer, 1981).

The purpose of teaching about human rights in a nursing course is to develop skills in analysing critically the basic human rights that are our concern because of our responsibilities as health professionals.

Does your list of learning objectives include:

- developing an awareness of own rights and the rights of others;
- raising own consciousness concerning the human rights of groups who need to have their rights defended;
- becoming sensitive to human rights as a humanizing element in nursing practice;
- sharpening critical skills in analysing human rights;
- preparing to teach about human rights?

ACTIVITY

Although the aim of your session is to assist students to analyse human rights and to sharpen their critical skills rather than to teach a subject, you will need to have a working knowledge of human rights as well as skills in managing the sessions. How will you prepare for a session on human rights?

FEEDBACK

- Get to know what your students know (or don't know). Singer (1981) speaks with some authority as a teacher and writer on human rights. In his view, a considerable percentage of the university students he teaches seem unaware of the existence of disadvantaged groups in the community. There is a strong possibility that nursing students are more aware because of their contact with health care, but they may also have 'blind spots' to other areas of disadvantage in the wider community.
- Be aware of the role of the ombudsman in your city and have a working knowledge of the human rights problems that your ombudsman deals with.
- Read about: the doctrine of human rights in such general texts as Kamenka and Tay, 1981; human rights in health professional education and practice (Purtilo, 1983); human rights and nursing (Benoliel, 1983; Thompson, Melia and Boyd, 1988; Johnstone, 1994).
- Remember that your human rights session is primarily a consciousness-raising session to prepare your students for their role in recognizing the rights of patients and in assisting patients to understand the implications of those rights, e.g. giving informed consent to treatment.
- Resist the urge to prepare your session as if it were a mini-lecture on human rights. First, you risk the charge of moralizing because you will find it hard to avoid advocating a set of values, which could be at variance with your students' and belongs in the values-clarification sessions. Second, the aim of the session is for the student to engage in an analysis of human rights and to reflect on or work through the issues involved. This expectation implies that the teacher also works through the issues with the students. This is a clear indication to students that human rights is not a specialized

subject to be learned but a way of thinking and behaving. As a role model of an analyser and critical thinker you are enabling the student to observe and work with a real person.

- Become skilled in identifying fallacies in analysing human rights arguments. Listen to live debates on radio; attend community meetings on local rights issues; read the report of a skilled analyst. Study the steps in moral reasoning: general (Phenix, 1966; Fenner, 1980) and nursing (Aroskar, 1980; Purtilo, 1983; Thacker, Pring and Evans, 1987; Thompson, Melia and Boyd, 1988; Rumbold, 1993; Johnstone, 1994).

INVOLVING YOUR STUDENTS IN HUMAN RIGHTS ISSUES

Purtilo's article (1983) gives a summary of the morals and norms appropriate to the health professions:

- **Duties:**
  - do no harm;
  - be faithful to contracts;
  - do all one can for the patient.
- **Rights:**
  - of patients;
  - of health professionals;
  - of society.
- **Responsibilities:**
  - of health professionals;
  - of patients;
  - of society.
- **Justice:**
  - seek a fair distribution of resources;
  - compensate for injuries.

ACTIVITY

Adhering to these duties, rights, responsibilities, and conditions of justice constitutes the moral dimension of the delivery of health care. While that may well be true, what exactly does it mean? How can the teacher use the framework for analysing human rights?

FEEDBACK

Kamenka and Tay (1981), and other workers in the same volume, stress the importance of considering human rights in their context, not as an abstraction in a vacuum. In choosing an universal right for analysis in your session it is important to set it in its context so that students will be able to relate easily to the problem.

Take, for example, the right of dissent, set in the context of a whistle-blower who has reported theft of equipment from a community centre and who as a result has lost her job. Stereotyped positions on this issue are likely to come to the minds of students as 'the community' and in turn community centres represent collective rather than personal responsibility. For example, such assertions as the following are frequently heard.

- Whistle-blowers are just trouble-makers.
- It's OK if the stuff's not needed, isn't it?
- It belongs to the community, doesn't it?
- Some people just wait for a chance to 'put others in'.
- It's not worth the trouble to report anything like that.
- Whistle-blowers should be supported.

and so on.

Instead of individual students taking a position, two groups could prepare to face each other with prepared arguments for dealing with a series of human rights problems. The strategy resembles a debate but the teacher's role is not as an adjudicator but a clarifier of views, facilitator of critical analysis and supporter of students caught in the cross-fire of contentious debate.

Other examples that could be used are:

- fair distribution of resources among acute care, preventive care and age-related distribution;
- informed consent – patients' rights;
- quarantine of HIV/AIDS people to protect the community from infection;
- resuscitation of people over 70 years of age.

HUMAN RIGHTS AND NURSING PRACTICE

As your students gain skill in analysing human rights issues, and depending on their level of maturity and their experience in nursing and health care, you and your students will want to move the sessions more into the realm of nursing practice. There is value in beginning with issues outside the field of nursing rather than moving immediately into nursing issues with junior students who lack sufficient experience and whose relationships with patients needs to grow 'naturally', person to person, in the beginning stages of their learning to nurse. So many pressures – unfamiliarity and inexperience; stress resulting from the severity of illness or death of patients, emergencies and crises – fill a new student's experience and require time to work through.

The issue for teachers is to encourage the skills of constructive critique and to anticipate the amount of support students may need during vigorous discussion.

On the other hand, extending the human rights concept from community issues, student issues and finally to patient's rights through a series of experiential strategies has the effect of drawing on the students' personal knowledge and individual values and expanding their understanding to an appreciation of shared values of peers, societal values and eventually to professional values and ethics.

NURSING ROLES AND HUMAN RIGHTS

ACTIVITY

What roles in nursing or nurse education would you consider important to examine in terms of their opportunity for recognizing and defending human rights in health care and education?

FEEDBACK

It would be hard to omit any direct contact role of nurse and patient, or teacher and student, as the basic principle is that human rights are fundamental to harmonious relationships. The dehumanizing potential of technological and bureaucratic routines is a threat to all of the participants. Nevertheless, there are some roles specially selected by nurses because of their heightened awareness of human rights issues or because their previous training and experience singles those nurses out as particularly suited to acting in such a role. For our purposes it is useful to analyse the role and to involve students in realizing its implications.

For example, some of these roles are:

- patient advocate;
- change agent;
- academic counsellor;
- consumer activist;
- student union officer;
- community liaison developer.

ACTIVITY

You have decided to involve your senior students in a session aimed at:

- examining the human rights aspects of these roles;
- analysing the issues involved for patients, nurses, students and teachers.

How would you structure the session so that your aims were reached?

FEEDBACK

If you are a confident discussion leader you could choose to guide the students through a free-ranging discussion. The issues certainly lend themselves to fruitful discussion and the guides to managing small groups in Chapter 4 will assist you to draw the group's discussion to conclusions. However, constraints of time and class size often demand a structure that allows maximum opportunity – for each student to be involved. A suggested structuring you could try for a 2-hour session is:

After a brief introduction to the session (5–10 minutes):

1. Distribute the roles of patient advocate, change agent and so on, so that each small group (or individual students or pairs if your group is very small) is assigned a role.
2. Provide a brief human rights problem on, for example:
   - informed consent;
   - access to information;
   - right of choice;
   - freedom from discrimination;
   - freedom from harassment;
   - self-determination;

   and introduce the task (5 min).

3. Give each group the task of drawing up a list of responsibilities of the incumbent of the role so that the rights of the persons they were most likely to serve were protected (allow approximately 30 min).
4. Without returning to the large group for discussion, the second task for the group is to draw up a list of rights for their respective client, patient or students (allow approximately 30 min).
5. Merge the groups, i.e. patient advocate and change agent, consumer activist and liaison developer, academic counsellor and student union officer, to provide comparison of the 'bills of rights' (15 min).
6. Returning to the large group, discuss the issues involved for students, teachers, patients and clients through group reports and a summary of the rights identified by the groups (20 min).

HUMAN RIGHTS IN SPECIFIC SITUATIONS

A useful strategy to use as a summarizing session is a series of trigger films. Careful choice of the triggers to exemplify the increasing complexity of human rights problems and to move from students' problems to patients' problems is important. You could use, for example, trigger films such as the following.

* A student asks the teacher for justification of the marking scheme in a recent examination and why his result was 'fail'!
* A patient refuses to take medication offered by the nurse.
* A patient and a nurse seek clarification of a proposed extensive surgical procedure.

Nichols, Beeken and Wickerson (1994) describe a trigger film that could be used for discussion of ethical issues such as withholding information from a patient; the patient's right to know; the nurse as patient's advocate.

If trigger films are not available, the scenes could be acted out in role play, but the advantage of trigger films is their capacity to sharpen the involvement of students and to rivet their attention. Usually the vignette is sufficiently short for the issue portrayed to be left without a suggested outcome. Before each vignette the students are asked:

* to imagine you are the nurse (or student);
* what would you say or do?

and to record their responses following each vignette.

Students' responses are usually immediate and very revealing of the strength of their reactions (sometimes even to their own surprise). What they would say or do in the confidential circumstances of the classroom (before the reaction is thought through for its social approval) gives an indication of underlying beliefs and values. Sharing their responses in a small supportive group can extend students' understanding of the human rights at issue. Also having the opportunity of coming to grips with their own response and affirming or analysing it is in itself a humanizing experience.

In summary, the purpose of teaching about human rights is to introduce students to a way of thinking about their responsibilities as individuals, citizens and health professionals in preserving and fostering an acceptable set of behaviours (morals or norms) for living and working peacefully and harmoniously together (Purtilo, 1983).

Another strategy is to give students a number of stereotyped responses of people to a problem, such as the withholding of nutrients from dying patients. Each student then takes a position on the stereotypes and defends it. After the group's discussion and the teacher's prompting, an analysis of each position can be achieved. The aim is for students to analyse their comments and to identify the presuppositions that form the basis of their beliefs. For the teacher, the role taken is one of clarifying the students' views, pointing out inconsistencies and leading students towards an understanding of moral reasoning. Examples from clinical practice are, unfortunately, not hard to find, and the students themselves could suggest examples from their own experiences as citizens in the community as well as learners in clinical practice.

Other examples: euthanasia; requiring quarantine for HIV/AIDS people to protect the community; patients as subjects for experimentation; the exploitation of patients as 'clinical material' for student learning

NURSES AND ETHICAL DECISION-MAKING

The purpose of teaching ethical analysis and decision-making is to provide for reflective thinking and through such thinking to identify the guidance necessary in resolving ethical problems. Your students in a course of nursing ethics (preceded by values clarification and discussions on human rights) will no doubt come to these sessions with an expectation that there will be learning materials to assist their reflective thinking. In an important sense, therefore, what has been covered by the previous sections represents preparation for learning about the complex skill of ethical analysis and decision-making.

Hunt (1992) points to the inclusion of ethics in nursing courses as a way of leading health care 'out of its technocratic impasse and point medicine and management in a greener and more democratic direction' (p 323). He further supports encouragement rather than suppression of the 'criticisms and uncertainties that come with an (ethics course)' (p 323) and cautions that there is 'a risk that lecturers who have probably been influenced by one or two bio-ethics texts or a crash course from a bio-ethicist, will relay to students inappropriate or garbled ideas and methods'.

As we saw in the last section of this chapter, adhering to duties, rights, responsibilities and fairness is part of the moral dimension of health care. Purtilo (1983) defines the terms 'morals' and 'ethics' neatly: 'Morals are the content of ethical reflection. Ethics is a discipline designed to sort out conflicts among duties, rights or responsibilities. Therefore, ethics analyses problems involving morals.'

Explaining the basis of ethical analysis Purtilo continues: 'It is useful to think of the moral norms described above (duties, rights, responsibilities, justice) as "elements" of ethical analysis. These elements can be observed, weighed, assessed and compared when they conflict.'

Although sometimes in critical situations there is no opportunity for reflective thinking or for weighing all the elements – rather, an immediate action is required (for example, triage) – preparation for exercising such a responsibility lies in a careful consideration of the steps involved during a well planned learning session.

The philosopher and educator Phillip Phenix states: 'The realm of ethics then, is right action. The central concept in this domain is obligation or what ought to be done. The "ought" here is not an individual but a universal principle of right' (Phenix, 1966).

So when a health worker asks 'What ought I to do in this situation?', the question calls on more than a clarification of values and human rights but, in addition, draws on ethical principles and theories in order to reach a resolution. Obviously, the skill involved is complex and although there are 'tools' to use, it seems preferable to continue an emphasis on the 'way of thinking'. Use of a tool implies some control or power over an object or a situation. What we are implying is really the opposite of a technology; it is the use of imagination, concern, compassion and intellect in the application of a universal principle in order to arrive at a moral solution that will be in the best interests of the person(s) involved.

In *Bio-Ethics, A Nursing Perspective*, Johnstone (1994) points to a clear demarcation of nursing ethics from other categories of bio-ethics.

> Bio-ethics, in essence, is a sub-class of ethics, which, in turn, is a branch of philosophy. Medical ethics and nursing ethics, on the other hand, are distinctive specialized fields of inquiry naturally

born of the practices of medicine and nursing respectively. Although the facts and concerns of these two disciplines overlap in many areas, they are ideologically separate in their endeavours, and it would be conceptually incorrect to treat them as being synonymous.

(Source: Johnstone, 1994, p 38)

Johnstone's (1994) position can be graphed as shown in Figure 7.1.

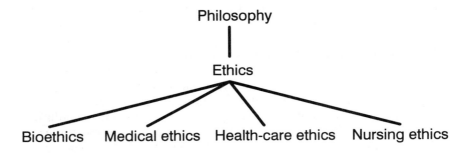

Figure 7.1   Ethics graph.

There is support for the distinctively separate disciplinary approach to ethics taken by Johnstone. For example, *Issues and Ethics in the Helping Professions* (Corey, Corey and Callanan, 1993) has been written for counsellors and social workers to examine specific areas where ethical analysis is required in their day-to-day work.

Most professions have ethical codes that are specific to their area of practice. It is important to realize that, as Figure 7.1 depicts, each of the disciplines draws its ethical knowledge and principles from the same source, i.e. from the discipline of ethics. The value of each profession introducing its learners to the rights and responsibilities of both the client or patient and the health professional, and to the process of dealing with ethical conflicts, cannot be argued. In fact, an ethical approach often demands that a number of disciplines are involved in discussion and resolution.

ACTIVITY

What do you want your students to achieve by the end of your sessions in ethical decision-making?

FEEDBACK

Naturally, the level of students in the course and their clinical experience would be taken into account, but by and large, you could expect the following:

- first, competence in analysing an ethical problem;
- second, skills in applying the steps in ethical decision-making to resolve an ethical dilemma.

Competence in analysing an ethical problem

An ethical problem may arise out of everyday situations such as keeping a promise, honouring a contract to produce an outcome, completing a treatment or an assignment, or explaining the concept of informed consent so that satisfaction that the patient has understood has been achieved before the document is signed.

Some ethical problems border on legal problems. An example is failing to honour an agreement about the care of a patient and thereby incurring a charge of negligence. Legal decisions are therefore called for. However, ethical problems are not dispensed with by a legal decision when an analysis of the situation reveals that an ethical dilemma exists.

A series of questions has been devised to analyse an ethical problem (Hynes, 1980, p 20) which, in brief, are as follows.

- What is the medical/nursing problem and the corresponding ethical question?
- Who is involved?
- What is the role of each individual involved?
- Am I the decision-maker for either the clinical problem or the ethical issue?
- Having reviewed alternative courses of action, what are the implications of any decision for myself, and those identified as being involved?
- Does this decision reinforce my general value orientation?

Skills in applying the steps in ethical decision-making to resolve an ethical dilemma

Ethical dilemmas are the most perplexing of ethical problems as they involve inter-relationships in which there are conflicts and tensions. Bioethical dilemmas arise in health care when a choice has to be made between two equally unattractive alternatives. Purtilo (1983) warns that the health professional involved should make certain that it is an ethical dilemma before acting to resolve the situation, as the implications for the patient and the health professional of hasty decisions are grave.

A four-step process of analysis is advocated: 'The health professional must ask:

- Do I have all the relevant data I can get about this situation?
- What kind of moral problem is this?
- What are my alternatives for responding?
- In the end, what can and should I do to alleviate or attenuate the distress caused by the problem (Purtilo, 1983).

A moral (or ethical) decision-making model which reflects the nursing process is advocated by Johnstone (1994, p 183). This involves:

- assessing the situation;
- diagnosing or identifying the moral problem;
- setting moral goals and planning an appropriate moral course of action;
- implementing the moral plan of action;
- evaluating the moral outcomes of the action implemented.

Johnstone's model is presented diagrammatically as a circular process in Figure 7.2.

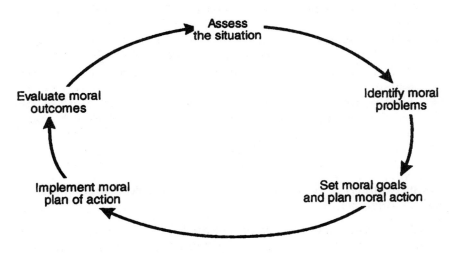

Figure 7.2   Ethical decision-making model.

A detailed hypothetical patient with a diagnosis of cancer is presented by Johnstone (p 184–191), showing how the decision-making model could be applied.

ACTIVITY

You have decided to use the Johnstone model in your class of undergraduate students. What strategies could you use so that students would gain experience in identifying and resolving ethical problems?

FEEDBACK

Students are often confronted by ethical issues in their clinical practice. Ask them to bring an example to class, preferably a dilemma which is yet to be resolved and in which a decision has to be made between alternatives neither of which will result in a desirable outcome.

Working in small groups, using the Johnstone model, the following steps could be facilitated by the teacher:

Steps	Process
1. Assess the situation	Students suggest all relevant sources of information in addition to the nursing problem
2. Identify moral problems	Students weigh up the moral obligation, rights and duties involved and decide whether a dilemma exists
3. Set moral goals and plan moral action	Students discuss who should decide; what values are involved; whose values; whose rights; what consequences follow a decision to act in one way or another; what ethical theory could assist the decision
4. Implement moral plan of action	Decide a strategy for carrying out the decision
5. Evaluate moral outcomes	

Choices and conflicts have arisen in issues such as prolongation of human life through the advent of life-support systems, increased knowledge of genetics and genetic engineering, increased sophistication in clinical research, *in vitro* fertilization and judgement about human life such that ethical decisions in health care are rising in complexity and frequency.

The steps in resolving ethical dilemmas have been variously described by Curtin (1978) and Aroskar (1980). Curtin's model includes the factors of background information, identification of ethical components and ethical agents, identification of options, application of principles and resolution. Aroskar's model for analysing an ethical dilemma consists of three elements: data base, decision theory dimensions, and ethical theories and positions. The analysis of an ethical problem is traced by Aroskar in *Anatomy of an Ethical Dilemma* (1980), showing how each step in the model is applied.

The difference offered by Curtin (1978) and Aroskar (1980) from the steps advocated by Hynes (1980), Purtilo (1983) and Johnstone (1994) is the important addition of the application of ethical theories in order to resolve the dilemma.

ACTIVITY

In achieving competence in analysing an ethical problem what skills would you expect of your students?

FEEDBACK

By this stage, having proceeded from values clarification and human rights considerations, you would be looking for indications that your students could:

- identify the difference between value judgements and judgements based on evidence;
- recognize and state their own biases;
- question critically the basis on which historical decisions in ethical problems have been made;
- read scholarly articles on bioethics and professional ethics and discuss the issues involved;
- scrutinize the moral or ethical implications of the ethical position taken in the readings;
- apply their own insights in the analysis of ethical problems.

ACTIVITY

What learning strategies will you prepare to enable your students to achieve the objectives and to become competent in the skills listed above?

FEEDBACK

Resolving a bioethical dilemma is rarely the responsibility of an individual health professional. The interdisciplinary nature of bioethical issues means that the nurse needs to understand the issues from a number of perspectives and to use the various perspectives in the analysis of ethical issues.

In addition to the skills in the previous list, you would probably expect that the students could:

- develop an adequate framework for decision-making;
- recognize through studying ethical decisions the practical consequences of the theoretical convictions they hold;
- recognize the conflicting rights in particular ethical dilemmas;
- debate the need for a systematic ethical analysis in bioethical dilemmas;
- discern the role of creative imagination in providing alternatives before a decision is made in resolving an ethical dilemma;
- appreciate that ethical decisions demand a maturity able to accept the ambiguity, implications and consequences of decisions.

ACTIVITY

In applying the steps of ethical decision-making to resolve an ethical dilemma, what skills would you expect of your students by the end of your sessions?

FEEDBACK

The observations or experiences of ethical conflicts that students can bring to a discussion provide an effective learning resource. Encourage students to collect examples from newspapers that have an ethical component, or provide vignettes from your own experience. Regardless of the learning strategy used or whatever model of analysis is applied, it is important to select issues that are appropriate to the students' level of experience.

Wilson-Barnett (1986) describes three clinical vignettes which are accounts of ethical dilemmas faced by nurses within the complexity of multidisciplinary clinical practice.

One of these brief accounts is quoted below:

A 40-year-old lady was found to have a malignant breast lump and her consultant recommended mastectomy. Grief and dismay was evident to all as she wept for most of her first night in hospital and the following day. The ward sister tried to console her for over 2 hours on that morning. Surgery was scheduled for the next day and a nurse was assigned to her care that evening and for the next morning. By the evening the patient was discussing her diagnosis and treatment, albeit tearfully. She asked about the possibility of other treatment and the nurse suggested that she discuss this with the doctor before signing her consent form. By the time the house surgeon arrived to explain the procedure it was 8 o'clock that evening and he was rather shocked by the patient's bevy of questions and tried hard to explain why mastectomy was the best treatment. When he left the patient he expressed his anger at this unexpected turn of events to the nurse, whom he reprimanded for encouraging the patient to doubt the prescribed treatment.

The nurse in this case became very tearful and said she believed she had done what was best for the patient, who had clearly wanted more information. She also explained that she considered informed consent implied the right of the patient to ask questions about alternative treatments. This conversation did not allay the house surgeon's irritation and he then complained about the nurse to the ward sister, who duly reprimanded her the next day.

(Source: Wilson-Barnett, 1986)

Discussion of vignettes such as this, where students are guided in analysing the nursing and ethical problems, provide rich learning experiences. The availability of a multidisciplinary team, including an ethicist, during the discussion would increase the benefits to students, patients and health care. 'Nursing and medical education should surely include more joint discussion sessions on ethical and treatment issues and be designed to provide more understanding of the principle and processes involved in providing the best and most complementary contributions to patient care' Wilson-Barnett (1986, p 126).

Another example of a teaching/learning strategy is described by Pederson, Duckett and Maruyama (1990). 'Structured controversy' is an interactive learning strategy where students in small groups resolve conflicts by learning skills of arguing for and against a specific position where there is disagreement. Because there is often conflict during the analysis of an ethical problem (such as euthanasia, abortion, whistle-blowing), Pederson, Duckett and Maruyama (1990) believe that there are potential benefits of conflict that students can gain through structured controversy. As such 'it serves as a rehearsal for dealing with future ethical problems' (p 153).

Plan for structured controversy

Question

Should students perform invasive techniques (i.v. injections) on patients or on themselves? Assume that no permission has been given by the unconscious patient and it is not known whether the veins are to be used for essential treatment later. Assume that the guidelines for professional practice are that i.v. injections must be practised and the competency assessed before graduation. Assume also that the examining clinical educator has been called to an urgent meeting and the i.v. injection has been drawn up by the student.

Objective

1. Present arguments for and against the student proceeding to give the i.v. injections.
2. Perform a critique on the validity of the arguments presented by others.
3. Defend your own position, against the critique of others, using rationale based on ethical principles and theories, law, nursing and medical knowledge and other relevant considerations.
4. Prepare a written summary of conclusions reached by the group, including rationale.

Task

Work co-operatively in groups of four to accomplish the objective above. You may want to consider the following factors, but do not feel limited by them.

•   Ethical issues

- Ethical principles
- Practical considerations
- Legal considerations
- Professional guidelines
- Personal beliefs and values
- Institutional policies and procedures
- Formal codes.

(Source: Adapted from Pederson, Duckett and Maruyama, 1990)

Reilly (1978) has proposed a 'dilemma worksheet' in the light of Kohlberg's (1972) theory of stages of moral development.

Davis and Aroskar (1978) and Davis and Krueger (1980) include resources from which learning materials can be structured.

Aroskar (1980) suggests a format of 'ethical rounds', similar to the case study method, where actual or hypothetical situations are analysed for their specific ethical dilemmas. Davis (1979) has also used ethical rounds successfully with intensive care nurses.

In summary, this chapter has dealt with the need to counteract the dehumanizing effects of technology in modern health care by sensitizing students to the values and human rights that affect daily decisions about the well-being of patients and families. The chapter also indicated the importance of including ethics in a nursing curriculum because of the fundamental (but complex) skill of ethical decision-making in which nurses and other health professions are involved to an increasing extent.

No doubt, as you have progressed through this chapter (which deals with the way values, human rights and ethics might be taught), you have questioned many of the assumptions on which the teaching methods are based. If that is so, the chapter will have worked in the way intended. There are often no clear right or wrong prescriptions to follow in teaching this area of nursing practice. Clearly, what works with one group may prove unsuccessful with another.

Teachers often find it helpful to pool their unsuccessful attempts at teaching as well as their achievements, so that they can draw upon their experiences in a productive way. This chapter is also a way of facing the values we, as teachers, hold in our commitment to seeking the most fruitful ways of assisting students to learn to nurse as independent individuals. 'The good news is that nursing ethics now serves nurses as professionals and persons more effectively than before. Instead of teaching silence and obedience, they now favour assertiveness, forthrightness, advocacy, excellence, and fairness for professionals and clients alike' (Haddad and Kapp, 1991).

ACTIVITY

After working through this chapter, what advantages do you see for students in a course of values clarification, human rights and ethics? What challenges for the teacher have come to mind?

FEEDBACK

Values clarification

Challenges for the teacher

- Values clarification could suggest that students are free to choose any set of values in health care, regardless of professional ethics.
- The method of values clarification may be treated superficially.
- It is time-consuming to teach.
- It is demanding of teaching skills.

Benefits for the student

- Values clarification provides students with a sense of assessing their own values and the values of others.
- It leads to values as a principle of action enables students to identify their reasons for preferring and prescribing one view over another.
- It sensitizes students to thinking about human rights and professional ethics.
- It emphasizes the valuing aspects of making judgements.

Human rights

Challenges for the teacher

- Human rights teaching is demanding of intellectual discipline.
- It is demanding of skills in examining issues of human rights and facilitating students' skills of critical thinking.
- It leads to examination of the issue of students' and teachers' rights.
- It could trap teachers into moralizing.
- It is often difficult to shift the emphasis for students from personal values to universal values.
- Human rights teaching could make teachers vulnerable to criticism because of lack of substantive content in the area of human rights.

- It is difficult to retain a focus on students' progress in critical thinking rather than a mastery of content as demanded by other areas of the curriculum.

Benefits for the student

- Human rights teaching draws on values clarification to explore the value conflicts in health care.
- It sensitizes students to the rights of disadvantaged groups.
- It raises issues of the responsibility of nurses to protect the rights of others and of themselves.
- It identifies the role of nurses in assisting patients and families to clarify their values, beliefs and rights.
- It enables students to examine the concept of rights and obligations.
- It assists students to clarify the different kinds of rights that exist.
- It prepares students for inter-professional discussion of patient rights in health care.

Ethics

Challenges for the teacher

- Teaching ethics presents a challenge to differentiate between the strategies of nursing process (problem-solving) and ethical decision-making (resolving an ethical dilemma).
- It could make teachers vulnerable to the charge of intellectualizing in place of experiencing ethical decision-making in the real situation.
- The ambiguous nature of ethical decisions could create insecurity.
- Constant support of students is needed, as ethical theories and strategies can only serve as a guide to resolving a dilemma; each situation requires personal inputs of intuition, experience, maturity and understanding.
- Support is also needed for students as they face the fact that rarely can a satisfactory resolution to an ethical dilemma be obtained. Choosing between two equally unattractive alternatives ensures that the final conclusion is less than desirable.

Benefits for the student

- Ethics teaching encourages critical thinking as a skill.
- It legitimizes time spent in reflective thinking.

- It extends the students' awareness of both the benefits of high technology and the drawbacks for individuals caught in dilemmas of accepting or rejecting the benefits.
- Learning the ethical component of nursing practice is pervasive and contributes to the students' personal knowledge and growth.
- It integrates ethical decision-making into day-to-day nursing skills.
- It leads to an open forum between health professionals.

Assessing learning 8

INTRODUCTION

Assessing student learning in the 1990s reflects the developments and trends in nursing education discussed elsewhere in this book. Holistic and caring philosophies, clinical decision-making, critical reflectivity and group problem-solving have been accompanied by a critical examination of assessment of student learning. Traditional assumptions have been questioned and innovative approaches to assessing many aspects of performance have been, and continue to be, developed. Assessment is no longer viewed as an unidimensional test of student ability but rather as a multidimensional part of the learning process. Devising methods for assessment which contribute to the students' learning has become a major component of the teacher's job.

When you have completed this chapter you should be able to identify the purposes of student assessment, to choose assessment strategies appropriate to those purposes and to plan and implement effective assessment procedures.

It will be useful to begin by clarifying three terms which are often used interchangeably – assessment, evaluation and examination. For the purposes of this chapter, 'assessment' is taken to mean the processes by which teachers attempt to gauge students' progress and learning; assessment may or may not involve quantifying that progress in terms of marks or grades. 'Evaluation' is reserved for the broader process of determining the effectiveness of the education students are receiving; assessment will contribute to evaluation but so may other processes such as observations of teaching, interviews and opinion surveys. 'Examination' refers to the formal mechanisms by which assessment is sometimes accomplished.

PURPOSES OF ASSESSMENT

As with most educational planning, the planning of assessment requires that you decide what you are trying to achieve before you embark on your planning exercise. Too often assessments are planned from the other direction – teachers start from the point of planning assessments to fit with the traditional pattern of their school: for example, end of term examinations or final examinations. A more rational starting point is from the consideration of the purposes of the assessment.

ACTIVITY

Think of the assessments which your students undertake. Make a list of the assessments, the times at which they are carried out, and the main purposes for which they are intended.

FEEDBACK

As a minimum, you have probably listed term tests, whose marks contribute towards final grades given to the student, and end of year or final examinations, whose marks determine whether students will be permitted to progress to the next stage of the course, to graduate or be registered to practise.

Until a few years ago this would have been an average schedule of assessments in many nursing schools. It fulfils the first main purpose of assessment which is to allow you to certify students as competent (in theory at least, but more about that later). These assessments have been called 'summative' because they represent the aggregate or final result of student learning. Such a limited schedule, however, neglects the other important purpose of assessment, which is to help students to learn. Of course it may motivate students to learn, but that is not the same as ensuring that their learning is usable and lasting (Chapter 3). Assessments used as a method to guide learning in progress have been called 'formative' because, by providing feedback on performance, they help the students to form or shape their learning in desired directions.

Assessments, used as contributors to learning, can achieve the following purposes.

- They can be more reliable in certifying competence if they are employed over a wide range of time and experience throughout the students' learning career to ensure that students are mastering the learning objectives as they proceed.

- They can help students to determine how well they are progressing and to estimate how much more work, and in which areas, they should concentrate on to reach an acceptable criterion.
- They can help the teacher to identify individual learning needs and to suggest remedial action.
- They can provide practice for students in self- and peer-assessment skills that they will need when they are practising professional nurses.
- They can encourage students to keep up to date with class work, rather than adopting the very ineffective strategy of 'cramming' at the last minute.
- They can help the teacher to determine how effective the course is.

The main thrust behind all of these purposes is that assessment can be used throughout the learning as a diagnostic aid and a source of feedback to both teacher and student. Contrast this with the more traditional approach, where assessment took place at the end of the course or unit of learning, where feedback was given to the student in the form of grades or marks and where the student had no opportunity or even specific information to enable her/him to make good the deficits in learning. In view of the fact that pass marks for such examinations were invariably considerably less than 100%, we can assume that significant numbers of nurses were able to graduate with significant gaps in their knowledge and skills and, worse still, no information about what those gaps were.

In response to this realization, a significant shift in the philosophy of assessment in the health professions has been the shift away from norm-referenced assessment towards criterion-referenced assessment. The move toward competency-based assessment is an example of an assessment system based on criterion-referenced assessment.

ACTIVITY

If you are familiar with the terms 'norm-reference' and 'criterion-referenced', take a few minutes to draw up a table which contrasts their main features. If you are not familiar with those terms, proceed straight to the feedback for this activity.

FEEDBACK

'Norm-referenced assessment' is the familiar process by which students are given marks and then graded according to their performance in comparison with other students in the class. Often, fairly arbitrary cut-off points are adopted for pass/fail or the award of honours. For example, an A grade might represent marks between 85% and 100%, a B grade might represent 70–84%, a C grade 55–69% and a fail might be less than 55%. Problems arise in this system from time to time when, for example, a whole class performs less well than expected, due perhaps to the characteristics of the examination, the teaching or the students. In any case, the faculty is faced with the decision either to fail a high number of students and award fewer A grades or to shift the pass-mark downwards. The latter is a regrettable choice in the health professions where schools are accountable for the safety of patients served by their graduates; however, it has been known to happen. The term 'norm-referenced' is derived from the fact that a graph of the distribution of student marks in examinations is usually normally distributed with the bulk of students achieving in the middle range and smaller numbers tailing off at each end of the curve as failures or distinctions.

Plainly translated, norm-referenced certifying examinations tell us that the faculty is satisfied to produce a small percentage of excellent students, a small percentage of failures and a majority of mediocre or barely competent students. After all, how certain can we be sure that the student who scores 56% and passes is more competent than the student who scores 54% and fails? The main justification for accepting this state of affairs has been that student ability is normally distributed and that examination performance reflects that innate ability and is therefore not amenable to teaching intervention.

Criterion-referenced assessment, by contrast, draws on the philosophy of mastery learning discussed in Chapter 3, in which it is suggested that, given appropriate teaching intervention, almost all students can achieve a high level of mastery – certainly in a tertiary level course in which students have been selected on the basis of their ability to begin with. Criterion-referenced assessment does not depend on comparisons among students, but on the extent to which each individual student is able to achieve the criterion set. Under ideal conditions the implication is that no students will fail and that all students will achieve 100% or very close to it. The normal curve no longer applies, and faculties that embark on this approach may find difficulty with their colleagues, who equate high pass rates with 'too easy exams' or 'soft options' and who may demand that students be graded for administrative purposes. Krumme (1975) and Bondy (1983) have provided good summaries of the case for criterion-referenced measurement in nursing. Sadler (1987) discusses the advantages and disadvantages of criterion-referenced assessment from the standpoint of general education.

A summary comparison table of the two forms of assessment is given in Table 8.1.

Table 8.1 Comparison of norm and criterion-referenced assessment

Norm-referenced assessment	Criterion-referenced assessment
Compares students with each other	Compares students with criterion
Easy to grade students	Difficult to grade students
Must provide uniform conditions of time, place and items	Uniformity not necessary – may be tested at any time
Assumes learning rates are equal	Allows for individual differences in rates of learning
Does not require definition of objectives and performance criteria	Specific learning objectives and performance criteria essential
Students unsure of what to learn	Students know exactly what is expected of them
Maintains dependence on teacher as arbiter of success	Develops self-direction and skills in self-assessment
May not ensure competence in essential areas	Ensures competence in essential areas
Does not provide specific feedback on mastery	Provides specific feedback on mastery of essential areas
Encourages competition between students	Encourages co-operation between students

You may now be convinced (if you weren't to begin with) that criterion-referenced assessment is a desirable goal for teachers in nursing to work towards. You might not be able to change all your assessment procedures overnight, so you should concentrate on identifying those areas of your subject which will most benefit from adoption of criterion-referenced and mastery-based learning experiences. Remember that, since students are not going to be graded on their performance in comparison with each other, you do not have to be concerned with secrecy of test items or providing uniform conditions to ensure fairness to every student. Each student is to be assessed individually on his or her merits and the conditions operating at the time of the assessment can be taken into account in deciding whether the student has achieved the criterion you would expect under those conditions. This means that criterion-referenced assessment can be an ongoing part of student learning, wherever that occurs, and that feedback is available to the student as often as is necessary for her/him to achieve the set criterion. Unfortunately, this very advantage also creates problems for the teacher and student if not handled correctly.

ACTIVITY

What problems do you envisage or have you experienced in the implementation of criterion-referenced assessment incorporating mastery-based learning? What solutions could be applied to those problems?

FEEDBACK

Problems and solutions in criterion-referenced assessment

A frequent problem is that, since criterion-referenced assessment can occur throughout the term or throughout the year in the form of progressive or formative assessment to provide feedback on progress, students begin to feel over-examined and constantly under stress. This problem applies particularly if the progressive assessments contribute to overall grading or marks. The climate that is essential for growth and skill development is lacking in situations where students fear revealing their uncertainties and deficiencies to their supervisors or tutors because they may be held against them in future assessments. Morgan, Luke and Herbert (1979) have pointed out that, especially in the clinical setting, students' achievement is too often evaluated while they are still learning. They advocate ensuring that teachers and students realize that there should be a time to learn and make mistakes that is distinct from the time to be evaluated. Simulations can be employed to ensure that the learning period of assessment is risk-free. Only when students have reached a satisfactory predetermined mastery criterion should they be assessed on their performance in the real situation and evaluated against the criteria for professional performance. Another variant of this solution is the establishment of a contract or understanding between students and supervisors which acknowledges the students' right to determine when assessment will take place. Students may be informally assessed by tutors or supervisors and provided with guidance and feedback on performance until the student, or the student and supervisor in conference, decide that the student is ready for formal assessment by another assessor. This strengthens the bond of trust and co-operation between student and supervisor and maximizes the student's opportunities to achieve mastery.

Mastery learning and criterion-referenced assessment can be very time-consuming and administratively difficult, given the likelihood that there will be considerable variation in the time taken for students to achieve the criterion level. Theoretically, students should have all the time and help that they need; however, in the real world this is rarely possible and teachers usually have to make decisions, based on their experience, about the maximum amount of time that a student can be allowed to persevere. Students who are markedly out of step with their colleagues should probably be counselled about their level of motivation to become a nurse, or personal problems that might be interfering with their learning efficiency. However, even within predetermined time limits, it is a challenging administrative exercise to ensure that all students are gainfully employed both before and after achieving mastery. Students who achieve mastery earlier can act as helpers to their colleagues, providing guidance and feedback and thus saving the teacher some time. This is usually a valuable experience for both students since they are developing skills in giving and receiving feedback from peers and the assistance given by one student to the other reinforces the 'teacher student's' knowledge and skills. Alternatively, faster students can be advanced to the next criterion task or can be given extra activities or responsibilities to extend their mastery of the topic. This approach also provides one solution to the dilemma of grading – extra credits towards advanced grades can be earned by students who contract to undertake activities beyond the basic mastery level. An approach to contract grading in clinical evaluation has been described by Schoolcraft and Delaney (1982).

One of the biggest advantages of criterion-referenced assessment also proves to be one of the biggest problems for some teachers, and that is the necessity to develop clear objectives for learning upon which criteria can be based. This invariably presents a number of dilemmas. It is necessary to be fairly specific in defining such criteria, otherwise they are useless – for example, 'demonstrates appropriate nursing behaviour' is an example of a criterion performance that is open to a wide variety of interpretation and is therefore unlikely to provide a reliable basis for assessment. A more specific behaviour might be 'demonstrates use of the nursing process in the approach to patient care'. A more specific criterion still would be 'demonstrates skills in assessing, planning, implementing and evaluating when offering nursing care to a hospitalized patient for whom the nurse has been given responsibility'. Of course we can go further still and probably keep going for quite some time in spelling out specific criterion behaviours within each of those skill areas of assessing, planning, implementing and evaluating. The teacher's problem becomes one of knowing where to stop. One of the dangers of specifying criteria is that, as competencies are broken down into more and more discrete subskills, we tend to lose sight of the overall picture, so that we run the risk of assessing students on their ability to perform discrete observable skills rather than to deliver effective care to the whole patient.

No one can give you the ideal answer to this dilemma of how specific to be in defining objectives and criteria because the need for specificity will clearly be greater in some circumstances than others. For example, junior nursing students will need more guidance about the component skills involved in phases of the nursing process, or in preparing a patient for surgery, or in relating to bereaved relatives; however, it can be assumed that senior students have mastered the basic skills and so assessment can be based on more holistic criteria such as the effective use of nursing process, the preparation – both physical and psychological – of patients for surgery and the empathic professional approach to bereaved relatives. At this level, according to Woolley (1977) 'Evaluation . . . is making a subjective judgement about the meaningfulness of the whole, both from the parts that are measurable, and from those that must be assessed intuitively'– the point being that we must also assess those aspects of nursing care which are not so easily reduced to specific components of observable behaviour.

Chapter 2 dealt, in some detail, with the process of defining learning objectives or outcomes. The remainder of this chapter will address the methods for translating those objectives into criteria for assessment.

METHODS OF ASSESSMENT

PLANNING THE ASSESSMENT PROGRAMME

Once you have decided whether you intend to use criterion-referenced or norm-referenced assessment and whether you intend to include formative as well as summative assessments in your programme you must then begin to ask yourself exactly what you wish to assess and exactly what methods will best enable you to assess those learning outcomes.

ACTIVITY

For the course that you teach, how do you decide what to include in assessments? Include both formative and summative assessments in your considerations.

FEEDBACK

What to assess

It has been suggested that student learning can be divided into three categories (Abbatt, 1992):

1. Must know
2. Should know
3. Nice to know.

Clearly, if you are interested in assessing student competence in essential criteria you will choose to assess the learning included in the 'must know' and also, ideally, in the 'should know' categories. On the other hand, if your main purpose is to obtain a broad spread of marks which will allow you to grade and rank students you will probably want to include a number of items which assess 'nice to know' learning to sort out those students who have exceeded the basic requirements. There is nothing wrong with adopting this approach: ranking of students is often necessary in order to award prizes or make employment decisions – however, 'nice to know' is no substitute for 'must know' and assessments in nursing should always ensure that essential performance criteria are assessed as an absolute minimum. Then, if there is time, energy and reason enough, students can be given the opportunity to demonstrate how far beyond their basic mastery levels they have been able to progress. Unfortunately, some examiners still concentrate on asking obscure or 'nice to know' information at the expense of 'must know' in the interests of producing a 'good discriminating test' rather than a good measure of competence. To illustrate, in a norm-referenced test the most efficient item is one which only 50% of students answered correctly; this is the item on which the test score variance is largest. Small variance lowers estimates of item reliability and variability. On the other hand, in a criterion-referenced test the most efficient item is one which most students answered correctly (Kirby, 1977).

If your assessment is intended to test mastery of 'must know' objectives, it naturally follows that students must know what those objectives are and therefore what they will be tested on. Some teachers object to this approach because they feel that students should not know what is going to be in the examination. Once again, this is an assumption that applies to norm-referenced rather than criterion-referenced assessments. If students are to be assessed on their mastery of set criteria there is no need for secrecy as there is if they are to be assessed for the purpose of ranking them against each other. Examinations are not supposed to trick or catch out the unprepared student, or to reward the student who is best able to 'psyche out' the hidden agenda of the teacher, but to provide a fair assessment of how well the students have learned what they are supposed to have learned.

In summary then, if you are committed to the mastery philosophy your assessment will include at least all these knowledge, skills and attitudes considered to be essential learning for nursing competence. If you prefer to remain with norm-referenced assessment your assessment should provide a sample of the field of knowledge, both essential and non-essential, which will enable you to discriminate amongst students based on the broad spread of their marks.

Formative assessment has an important role in criterion-referenced assessment, since it may be impossible to include all the essential performances in a single examination, or even a single series of examinations, at the end of the term, the year or the course. Assessments of mastery can be offered at appropriate points throughout the learning period and can be recorded to contribute to the final certification of competence. For example, assessments at the completion of clinical attachment periods can be used in this way.

The following checklist will assist you in planning your assessment.

1. Select the 'must know' and 'should know' objectives of your course.
2. Determine the knowledge, skills and attitudes components of those objectives.
3. Ensure that the level is appropriate – are you testing problem-solving or just recall of facts; are you testing skill components or holistic patient care?
4. Decide when would be the most appropriate time to assess each of these objectives. This will depend to a large extent on the structure of your course, but remember the importance of formative assessment and try to divide the course content into discrete units, which can be conveniently followed by tests of mastery of the unit objectives.
5. Decide what type of assessment would be most appropriate for each objective; for example, written tests can satisfactorily assess knowledge but procedural skills can only be effectively assessed in a clinical or simulated situation.
6. Within each type of assessment decide which format would best serve your purposes within your available resources; for example, would your knowledge objectives be best assessed by multiple choice, essays, short-answer questions or a combination of all of these?
7. Determine ways in which you will grade students if you require to do so. You could offer optional extra assessments or assignments, you could insert test items of greater difficulty, you could include some 'nice to know' objectives, you could determine weightings of marks on the basis of levels of objectives, or you could try offering students the opportunity to contract for higher grades.
8. Develop your assessment items or protocols and subject them to review by your colleagues. Do they meet the criteria for a good test – reliability, validity, feasibility? Will you need to train other assessors to ensure proper application of the assessment?
9. Check your final assessment programme to ensure that all essential competencies are represented and that you are assessing necessary higher order skills, attitudes and intellectual abilities rather than just knowledge.

Remember that, since all students aim to pass examinations, assessments exert a powerful influence on what students learn and the way they learn. Make sure that your examination questions are a good example of what you want the students to learn. If you do not test for essential skills then students are unlikely to bother to learn those skills properly.

SELECTING ASSESSMENT METHODS

There is a large variety of assessment methods, many of which you will be familiar with and will have used on many occasions. Some newer methods, however, are worth a closer look and some of the older methods you have been using could perhaps be used more effectively. A number of comprehensive books on assessment in general, and assessment in the health professions and nursing specifically, are available (Adkins, 1974; Morgan and Irby, 1978; Schneider, 1978; Katz and Snow, 1980; Neufeld and Norman, 1985; Battenfield, 1986; Garbin, 1991) so it is intended in the following to provide an overview of the major considerations involved in choosing assessment methods with specific references for more detailed aspects.

ACTIVITY

The following are some of the 'must know' objectives from your course. What method would you use to assess performance in each area?

1. Students must be able to recognize the clinical features of myocardial infarction.
2. Students must be able to record an accurate history and assess the nursing care needs of a patient admitted to the coronary care unit.
3. Students must be able to develop a nursing plan for the care of a patient admitted to the coronary care unit.
4. Students must be able to correctly set up the cardiac arrest trolley.
5. Students must be able to assist in the emergency management of a patient with cardiac arrest.
6. Students must demonstrate care and concern for the well-being of patients in their care and consideration for the needs of the relatives of seriously ill patients.

FEEDBACK

The first important thing to note about this activity is that most of the objectives cannot be satisfactorily assessed using only one method. Nursing performance is multidimensional and requires a variety of methods to adequately assess competence.

ASSESSING KNOWLEDGE

For convenience, we will consider the knowledge components of objective 1: 'Students must be able to recognize the clinical features of myocardial infarction'. Knowledge is an important component of clinical performance and assessment of knowledge is a necessary but not sufficient step in the assessment of competence.

For recognition of myocardial infarction, students would need to be able to list the clinical features of myocardial infarction or describe the typical appearance of a patient with myocardial infarction. There are a number of methods you could have chosen to assess this objective. Most commonly used methods would be as follows.

Short-answer questions

Short-answer questions would be appropriate here because the answer you are expecting could be easily covered in a few lines and would be easy to mark. The student's score could be based on the number of diagnostic features stated correctly in the answer. An example of a short-answer question would be: 'List five clinical features which would lead you to suspect that a patient has suffered a myocardial infarction' or 'Describe the typical clinical presentation of a patient who is suffering an acute myocardial infarction.'

Short-answer questions are a convenient way to test recall of information because they are quick to complete and to mark and therefore allow you to set a large number of questions, which sample a broad area of knowledge. Their disadvantage is that they encourage students to learn lists of facts that are easily and quickly recalled, rather than to learn underlying principles and to develop the habit of thinking things through.

Multiple choice questions (MCQs)

MCQs could be appropriate here because the question is factual and requires little explanation by the student. There are a number of different types of MCQ (see Anderson, 1981 and Kirby, 1982 for examples), but the most common and easiest to mark is the 'one from five', so called because the student is required to choose one correct response from five possible alternatives. An example of this type of MCQ is:

A 55-year-old man is brought to the emergency clinic with the story that he has collapsed in the street. He is pale, sweaty, has a weak, rapid irregular pulse and is breathless. Among his personal effects is a bottle of glyceryl trinitrate tablets. The most likely cause of his collapse is:

a) asthma
b) ruptured aorta
c) acute myocardial infarction
d) stroke
e) pneumonia.

Actually it is very hard to write a good MCQ item for an objective such as this because it is difficult to find sufficient distractors (incorrect alternatives) that are realistic enough to test the students' knowledge. The above MCQ is likely to be a very easy one answered correctly by almost all of the students.

Another commonly used MCQ is the true/false type:

Acute myocardial infarction:

a)	is always accompanied by chest pain	T	F
b)	may give rise to arrhythmias	T	F
c)	gives rise to symptoms of shock	T	F
d)	causes T wave inversion on ECG	T	F
e)	is fatal in 70% of cases.	T	F

Once again such items are difficult to write because there are few absolutes in nursing practice. Only a very naive student would agree with a question that includes the words 'always' or 'never'. Sometimes performance in MCQ tests is an assessment of how 'test-wise' the students are rather than how much they know.

The advantages of MCQs are that they are fast to answer, fast to mark and reasonably objective; i.e. they do not rely on individual judgements by examiners but have a predetermined set of correct answers, which can be marked by computer if necessary. These advantages are balanced, however, by the fact that good MCQs (those which are not ambiguous, not too easy or not too hard, or don't give too many clues or too few realistic alternatives) are very time-consuming to develop. For this reason, teachers often keep a bank of MCQs which have been shown to be good ones and which are used from year to year. The development of good MCQ items and tests, the analysis of item performance and the interpretation of student performance is a complex process which involves statistical manipulation. If you intend to use MCQ examinations you would be well advised to consult with your local educational testing service or to refer to the many detailed texts available.

The disadvantage of MCQs is that they provide all the necessary information and students need only recognize the correct information. Recognition requires even less thinking than recall and it encourages students to learn patterns of symptoms and lists of facts that can be learned at a glance. MCQs can be written to test problem-solving skills by, for example, providing a case history in the stem and a sequence of items that requires students to make progressive steps towards solution of the clinical problem (see Joorabchi, 1981 and Kirby, 1982). However, there are probably better ways to assess problem-solving skills and some of these will be dealt with later in this chapter.

Essay questions

Essay questions are less appropriate for a purely factual response because they are difficult and quite time-consuming to mark. For testing factual knowledge, essay questions have no advantage over a series of short-answer questions.

Oral examinations

Oral examinations are an extremely inefficient and ineffective way to test students' factual knowledge. They are time-consuming and they are not standardized so that different students may be asked questions in different ways and their responses judged according to the impressions of the examiner rather than by some predetermined criteria established by the teacher. In addition, many students find oral examinations very stressful and fail to perform well even though they may know quite a lot of factual material.

Uses and limitations of knowledge-assessment methods

What we have said about the knowledge component of objective 1 also applies to the knowledge component of objective 4 – students could be asked to list the items on the cardiac arrest trolley in a short-answer question or to identify the correct items in a multiple choice question.

Similarly, basic knowledge required in history taking (objective 2) could be assessed by asking the student to write a list of the questions they would ask, while in objective 5 they could be asked to write a brief description of the role of the nurse in the management of a cardiac arrest or to choose the most appropriate options from a multiple choice series of alternatives in response to a specific scenario in the question stem. However, objectives 2, 4 and 5 imply much more than simple knowledge: they also imply that the student will apply that knowledge to the various nursing responsibilities. It is not sufficient to ascertain that students know what should be done; it is important to make sure that they actually do what needs to be done at the appropriate times, in a manner which is consistent with good nursing care.

Assessing group projects

A problem associated with group projects is how to assess the individual performance of members of the group. What is it that individual students have actually learned? The question is particularly pertinent for programmes where the curriculum is based on problem-based learning. Group work is essential to the implementation of the programme. One method is to ask individual students to indicate, at the beginning of the project, the learning goal they wish to achieve during the group process. Assessment could then be based on the extent to which the goal had been reached.

Jacques (1984) advocates students keep a record of the work done for the group meeting as well as the work completed in the group. Two essays and three summaries of the students' own developing views over the period of a nine week course are required.

Gillette and McCollom (1990) evaluated the intellectual work of students in a course on group dynamics. Student behaviour in the group was ruled out for assessment as the influence of an assessment on group members' behaviour would obviously affect the dynamics of the group. The decision was to make the assessments similar to those in any other university course, that is, written papers. However the papers were handed in throughout the semester and were to relate events from the group sessions to concepts presented in lectures and readings. In other words, description and analysis as well as proposals for revisions in theory were expected.

ASSESSING CLINICAL PERFORMANCE

For the second objective listed on page 210 , recording a history and assessing the nursing needs of a patient, the student would have to demonstrate the ability to actually produce the history and assessment. The only real way to assess this is either to observe the student taking a history or to examine the written history and assessment which the student provides after spending time with the patient. The written product of the interview will tell you whether the student has obtained all the relevant information and been able to synthesize it in a meaningful way to formulate an assessment of nursing care needs, but it will tell you nothing about the spirit of the encounter or how well the student managed to establish rapport and develop a relationship with the patient. Direct observation or interview of the patient is an additional component which would have to be added to the assessment to provide information about the student's mastery of those relationship (or affective) objectives. We will leave consideration of the assessment of affective objectives for the moment and concentrate on assessment of skill performance.

Direct observation of skill performance can be arranged in a number of ways.

Formal clinical examinations

Clinical examinations can be set up and arrangements made for real patients from the wards or clinics to be present. Students may be left alone with the patient for a while, or the examiners may stay to observe all the students' performances. Facilities permitting, a desirable alternative could be to have examiners observing through a one-way window or on closed-circuit TV.

Of course it would be necessary for both student and patient to know that they were being observed but the lack of the actual physical presence of the examiner would probably enhance the interaction.

Objective-structured clinical assessment (OSCA)

Fahy and Lumby (1988) report the use of OSCA in a nursing programme after a search for a more reliable and efficient method than they had previously used. The assessment was not limited to psychomotor skills but included 'analysis of data, history-taking, problem identification, time management, attitudes, values and interpersonal skills – all essential components of effective nursing'.

The organization of the testing programme involved the setting up of 12 stations. At some, an assessor was present to observe a student actually performing. At others no assessor was present but the student watched a video trigger presentation or examined a slide or an X-ray and answered questions related to the display. Each student took 60 minutes to complete the examination and, as 12 stations were used, 12 students could be examined at the same time.

Student preparation for the examination commenced 3 weeks prior to the event. Sample vignettes (18 in all) were given to the students who were told that nine of them would form the basis of the OSCA activities. Teacher preparation consisted of a committee of six who wrote the exam. Each activity was reviewed for clinical significance, objectivity, structure, standardization of presentation and marking facility. Six additional teachers were trained to be assessors at various stations.

An example of an OSCA station with a short history of a woman aged 62 with pneumococcal pneumonia is given in the article. Activities include examining an X-ray and using the result to position the patient appropriately to drain the affected lung; performing percussion and vibration on a dummy and applying oxygen therapy. The activities test knowledge, interpersonal communication and psychomotor skills.

The authors include instructions and time allotted, marking criteria and the values attaching to each step in the activities.

The disadvantages of OSCA (or OSCE – objective-structured clinical examination) in terms of time needed for the assessment of complex skills, such as the ability to integrate information from a number of sources and whether the skill would be applied appropriately to a particular clinical problem, are discussed by Newble *et al.* (1994).

Assessment during clinical practice

It might be more appropriate for certain skills to be assessed during the course of the students' clinical experience. In-service assessment is appropriate for skills that are difficult to set up for a formal examination, such as assisting with a lumbar puncture, or skills that carry an element of risk and require close supervision, or just day-to-day skills and procedures such as lifting patients, presenting ward reports, etc., which need to be assessed but which are not necessarily part of summative assessment. Assessment during the course has been discussed earlier in this chapter, when it was emphasized that the distinction should be drawn between assessment to learn and assessment to certify.

Simulations

In some situations it is not desirable to assess students' performance with real patients or in real situations because of risk or discomfort or because the situation is not suited to examination conditions. Morgan, Luke and Herbert (1979) have described videotaped interactions and written case studies as simulations intended to assess students' ability to assess nursing care needs. Simulations also give more control over what happens in the assessment. For example, for the present objective different students may receive very different patients to interview and the amount of information they are able to elicit may not be entirely due to their skill in history-taking. Similarly some patients might present more straightforward problems than others and might be easier to assess. This is unavoidable because it would be unreasonable to expect the same patient to submit to several interviews by several different students. An alternative is to train simulated patients to provide a standard history, or for the examiner or teacher to play the role of the patient and provide the history. This latter method raises some problems if only one examiner is present because it is difficult to be both interviewee and examiner at the same time.

Infante (1985) devotes a chapter to simulations and their importance in clinical teaching and assessment. Simulations of clinical situations using videotaped vignettes have gained in popularity for evaluating basic nursing skills. Matthews and Veins (1988) used group video testing in an innovative testing programme. A group of students is recorded on videotape acting the parts of patient, student and evaluators. Prior preparation (5 days before testing) includes a brief scenario of a client. The group explores the situation and studies a list of performance criteria for the skills taught in the course. All students in the group must be prepared to play the roles of patient, student and evaluators, thus ensuring that preparation has included knowledge of assessment criteria as well as the nursing knowledge and skills demanded by the situation. The resulting tape contains the original client survey, nursing analysis, updated situation with assessment, nursing records and the students' group critique. Several faculty members view the tape and evaluate the performance using the same critical performance criteria used by the students. The authors claim that a holistic approach is used, the nursing process is applied and professional judgement occurs as students function in the simulated videorecording. It is interesting to note that, in addition to the holistic approach reported by the authors, students are still tested individually on nursing skills of safe practice.

Interactive video exams are used by the Regents External Degree Program in New York to evaluate the clinical learning of registered nurses (Lenburg and Mitchell, 1991). The assessment of student performance is based on outcome indicators.

Bersky and Yocom (1994) have accelerated assessment methods into the 21st century with computerized clinical simulation testing (CST). They envisage that 'It is conceivable that, early in the 21st century, a licensure candidate taking NCLEX-RN would receive a two-part examination. One part would include the administration of MCQs, via computerized adapted testing (CAT), and the second component would entail the administration of a series of CST cases to assess the ability to use nursing knowledge in simulations of client encounters' (p 125).

CST is different from interactive computer-based simulation programmes. There is no list of decision options to which the examinee is expected to react. Instead a brief introduction is given and then the examinee, using 'free text' entry, specifies the nursing actions she/he would take in the real situation. The authors foreshadow the use of CST as a teaching tool in education programmes and as a competency test for RNs rejoining nursing after a period of absence from active nursing. An evaluation of the scheme for nursing education in the USA will be undertaken in the 1993–1998 phase of the project. The results of the evaluation will be awaited with interest as computerized systems of living in the 21st century become a reality.

Observation tools

The two most commonly used tools for performance assessment in all these contexts are checklists and rating scales. Newble *et al.* (1994), after an extensive search of the literature, note that checklists and rating scales are commonly used where students' behaviour is observed and recorded as tests of performance. Checklists have higher observer agreement than rating scales. Longer checklists tend to be more reliable than shorter ones (p 217).

Checklists require the observer to judge whether certain behaviour has taken place. They are most effective where components of performance can be specified in detail (Katz and Snow, 1980). Checklists provide a list of detailed behaviours within a performance, sometimes in the sequence in which they should occur, and the observer is asked to record whether the behaviour was observed or not observed. A third option, such as 'not applicable', should be included. Because checklists are so detailed, they provide a useful profile of performance, which can be discussed with the student. If any essential component of the performance is omitted the student can be said not to have achieved mastery on that criterion and should be required to present for further assessment after more practice. Common important errors made by students should also be included so that the observer can note errors of commission as well as errors of omission.

It is possible to include considerations of attitudes and relationship skills in checklists for the observation of skill performance. Stecchi *et al.* (1983) have gone one step further in devising a clinical evaluation tool in the form of a checklist which can be applied in a variety of settings. They describe the tool as being organized around 22 objectives, which define the areas of clinical and theoretical competence the student is expected to achieve by the end of the junior year. To the right of each objective are four columns corresponding to the four clinical nursing courses. Each course column is subdivided into two additional columns designated 'S' for satisfactory and 'U' for unsatisfactory.

Checklists of discrete skills developed for a specific purpose, e.g. to meet the need of an objective State Board test for licensure, have been constructed from a behavioural-based model. Shifts in the philosophy of nursing practice have moved testing away from any suggestion of the testing of 'tasks' (Dunn, 1986). Emphasis on performance of a specific skill has sometimes resulted in beginning students being fixated on specifics rather than having a perspective on the patient as a whole (Matthews and Veins, 1988). Yet in the demonstration of a psychomotor skill it is still necessary to break the skill down into sequenced elements that the student can grasp in order to become technically competent as a beginning practitioner in the real world (Benner, 1984). There is of course, agreement that the criteria of 'action involving judgement' describes nursing activities and has led to a variety of clinical evaluation (not assessment) tools. Infante *et al.* (1989) comment that psychomotor skills remain the most commonly discussed issue in testing but have stimulated little research. The issue in testing is complex, involving objectivity and standards as well as the purpose of the test and the objectives of the course.

Rating scales require judgements by the observer about how well the performance meets the set criteria. Rating scales usually provide from three to seven options for the observer to quantify the level of performance of the student in comparison with an ideal standard. It is therefore important that the observers use a common standard. Some inexperienced observers make the mistake of rating a student nurse's performance against the standard they would expect of a graduate or experienced nurse. Assessors should spend time together identifying the standard to be used. A further problem with rating scales is that since they provide a means for quantifying the observer's judgements they provide a false sense of security. Numerical scores derived from rating scales can be just as subjective as unstructured opinions unless observers are trained to provide reliable (that is reproducible) judgements. Combining ratings from different observers can help to eliminate observer bias or unreliability. Rating scales are most appropriate to assess traits such as efficiency, judgement, ability to work with others (Irby and Dohner, 1976) and the ability to adapt to local characteristics and variations (Katz and Snow, 1980, p 32). Further examples of rating scales can be found in the references cited above under checklists.

Dunn (1986) describes the development of five scales for measuring the nursing skills of first-year learners and five for measuring the same nursing skills of second- and third-year learners (p 31). The tool is not used as an observation method as 'it cannot be used by watching the learner carry out isolated nursing tasks, it requires a working knowledge of their overall behaviour. It does in fact require continuing assessment. The assessors judge the learners' performance against ranked behavioural statements and not against a numerical level on a scale'. As the assessors use their own professional judgement it is difficult to see how the subjective nature of the measurement could be overcome.

The variety of formats possible is considerable. Cottrell *et al.* (1986) developed a rating scale to assign a letter grade to competencies of students based on the nursing process. A criterion-referenced rating scale was used. The tool was computerized, allowing students and faculty to evaluate student clinical performance every 2–4 weeks. An example of the tool is given in the article.

Remember that observers will need to be trained in the use of any rating scale that you choose or develop, and that baseline criteria for making the judgements should be explicit.

Other methods of assessing clinical performance

The anecdotal record

The anecdotal record suffers from the fact that it is anecdotal and that the information recorded may be unsystematic, unrepresentative of the student's behaviour in general and difficult to interpret for assessment purposes. The anecdotal record is often a mix of fact and opinion. Rines (1963) has suggested a standard format for recording anecdotal information which attempts to differentiate between fact and opinion – the anecdotal record should consist of three segments, a description of the context of the event, a description of the actual behaviour witnessed and only then a statement of the observer's opinion of the behaviour. Even when this approach is employed, however, there is difficulty in obtaining balance and spread of observations in relation to the objectives, and the information gathered is unlikely to be reliable enough for use in normative assessment, although it can be a useful approach to identifying students' problems in the formative context.

Hillegas and Valentine (1986) report a system of clinical assessment using daily anecdotal records. These are structured according to the five major clinical objectives of the course plus subobjectives for each particular course. A formative evaluation based on the anecdotal records is given to the students after each clinical placement. The need to assign a clinical grade at the end of the semester led to the construction of a rating scale to distinguish the range of grades from A to D.

The critical incident technique

The critical incident technique assumes that raters will make inferences about a person's general competence on the basis of the person's performance in a number of specific situations (Sims, 1976). In order that the data is generalizable, a number of general headings under which performance is to be assessed by grouping similar incidents must be established. In this way critical incidents can be used to develop a performance record based on core behaviours (Fivars and Gosnell, 1966). This approach fits well with criterion-referenced assessment where the core behaviours for mastery have been identified. Unfortunately there are logistic problems, which limit the usefulness of the technique, principally arising from uneven enthusiasm, interest and commitment among clinical staff who are expected to be reporters, and from the difficulties in establishing consensus on categories into which incidents fit. Dachelet *et al.* (1981) used critical incidents to obtain a holistic perspective, a broad picture of activities in a clinical practicum setting – they provide details of the categories and criteria used to classify incidents. Flanagan (1954) specified criteria for the use of critical incidents to assess clinical performance.

- The actual behaviour must be reported rather than general traits.
- The behaviour must be actually observed by the reporter.
- All relevant factors in the situation must be given.
- The observer/reporter must make a definite judgement of the 'criticalness' of the behaviour.
- The observer/reporter must make it clear why the behaviour is considered to be critical.

An example of a simple format for recording critical incidents is given in Figure 8.1.

Name of student: ....

Name of reporter: ....

Think of the last time you observed this student nurse do something that you thought was especially effective in contributing to patient care.

What led up to the situation?

Exactly what did the nurse do?

Why do you feel it was particularly effective?

Figure 8.1   Example of a format for recording critical incidents.

Trained observers can provide valuable data on performance using the critical incident technique and it can also be extended as a method for student self-reports, where students are asked to identify critical incidents in their learning experience and areas in which they need more assistance. Stainton (1983) has developed an alternative to critical incident recording which fits more easily with ward routine. A 'clinical experience record' for each student is kept in a loose-leaf binder in the ward and includes the following information:

- **assignment** – details of the patient;
- **learning experience** – including reasons why the particular assignment was chosen for the student, and the preparation necessary before undertaking the assignment;
- **nursing care planning** – anecdotal notations and evidence of preparation done for the assignment;
- **comments regarding implementation** – notations of how the student carries out the plan. Behavioural descriptions are recorded as objectively as possible.

The record provides a composite picture of experiences offered and allows progress to be reviewed with the learner.

ACTIVITY

In the light of what we have said so far perhaps you would like to reconsider the rest of the objectives on page 210. What methods would you use to assess the clinical performance objectives remaining in that activity?

3. Students must be able to develop a nursing plan for the care of a patient admitted to the coronary care unit.
4. Students must be able to correctly set up the cardiac arrest trolley.
5. Students must be able to assist in the emergency management of a patient with cardiac arrest.
6. Students must demonstrate care and concern for the well-being of patients in their care and consideration for the needs of the relatives of seriously ill patients.

FEEDBACK

A number of assessment methods are applicable to assessing clinical performance.

Developing a nursing plan could be assessed effectively by the critical incident or anecdotal record techniques or by the use of simulated patient encounters or even paper and pencil or computerized simulations.

Essay questions have been widely used to assess problem-solving skills but often the questions are not specific enough and students have to guess what the examiner wants them to write about. In addition essays are difficult to mark consistently – two different examiners may give quite different marks for the same essay unless they have agreed on some specific marking scheme which includes a list of the major points that should be covered in the essay. For this objective, however, a better method would be the modified essay question or MEQ (Knox, 1980). Modified essay questions are a series of short-answer questions which are related to a single clinical problem and which proceed from an initial scenario of the problem to its sequential development, progressively providing more information and requesting decisions from the student.

Since subsequent questions sometimes provide the answers to previous questions special measures must be taken in administering the test, for example, each page can be collected as the student finishes it and the next step in the problem given to the student. An advantage of the MEQ is that even if students answer a question wrongly, they do not necessarily lose marks for the whole MEQ. They can redeem themselves in the next section by realizing their error and progressing down the correct path. Marking the MEQ is also more reliable because essential points in each section can be defined as criteria. Discussion of the MEQ after the examination can be a learning experience that helps the students to develop a systematic approach to discussion of a clinical problem.

Setting up a cardiac arrest trolley is an excellent example of a performance that would be most effectively assessed by the use of a checklist, since it consists of a well defined set of observable behaviours which are easily specified and require little independent judgement by the observer.

Assisting in the emergency management of a patient with cardiac arrest could, theoretically, be assessed by observation in the real setting using a rating scale or critical incident format, but in practice it is very unlikely that such behaviours would be amenable to observation. The most feasible approach to assessing this very important objective is to assess theoretical knowledge in a written examination and to assess ability to apply that information in a realistic simulation in the nursing laboratory, where checklists, rating scales or other clinical performance observation schedules can be used to both assess and provide feedback to students on performance.

ASSESSING ATTITUDES

Demonstrating care and concern for patients and relatives is, of course, an attitudinal or affective objective which can only be assessed by direct observation of the student over a broad range of time and clinical experiences. Anecdotal records, critical incidents and rating scales all lend themselves to the assessment of affective objectives. There are a number of methods available for written assessments of attitudes such as semantic differential scales, questionnaires, self-reports (Girod, 1973; Oppenheim, 1966; Weinholtz and Stritter, 1982) and for simulated assessments such as responding to videotaped vignettes of events or people. These methods however suffer from problems of validity in that they demonstrate whether students know what the desired or appropriate attitudes are but they do not demonstrate that the student actually behaves according to those attitudes in the real situation. They are open to 'fakability' and to biases imposed by students providing socially acceptable responses.

There is always a value position inherent in attitudinal objectives and criteria and some teachers feel uncomfortable in asserting particular values or providing feedback to students whose values are not consonant with their own. Nevertheless, values are an integral part of nursing and must be taken into account in learning and assessment. Reilly (1978, p 63) clarifies the problem somewhat with the following statement: 'When students are asked for opinions, feelings, beliefs or points of view on value related issues, the opinion cannot be graded. However, the logic, accuracy and completeness of the rationale for the opinion can be graded.'

For example, students can be given a problem to solve which requires a choice on a value related issue and their responses can be judged on their ability to identify alternatives, predict consequences and provide a rationale for the preferred action. Essays would be an appropriate assessment method for this type of objective.

Attitudes, perhaps more than any other type of learning, require formative rather than summative assessment, and sensitive feedback where deficiencies are identified. Gordon (1978) has proposed a clinical model for assessment of student affect which recognizes this sensitivity. The basic components of the model are as follows.

1. Statement of affective objectives – begin with a general statement of the attitude and develop a narrative statement of a situation in which this attitude would be demonstrated.
2. Screen for potential behaviour problems to provide an early-warning system.
3. Clarify problems – involve the student and encourage self-assessment.
4. Assess specific behaviours and clarify whether differences from criterion are due to value differences or perception differences between student and adviser.
5. Provide assistance – joint planning, specific commitments to tasks.
6. Determine the potential seriousness of the problem.
7. If the problem has not responded to the above, formally inspect performance, with due notice to the student.
8. Take administrative action to suspend or dismiss if the student does not respond to the above measures and counselling.

ASSESSMENT OF REFLECTIVE PRACTICE

Since experiential learning has shown how to 'turn experience into learning' (Boud, Keogh and Walker, 1985) and since Schon's (1988) observations of the changes possible in health care through reflective practitioners, teaching for reflective practice has become an important component of nursing courses. The question for assessment is, should reflective practice be assessed and, if so, how could it be done?

Woolfolk (1989) notes that Schon's concept of learning reflective practice includes self-evaluation and evaluation from an 'expert' coach. The small, interactive personal programmes advocated by Schon raise philosophical and practical difficulties for the evaluation programme of nursing programmes. Woolfolk notes the traditional attitude of students (regardless of their discipline) to put learning energy into those subjects that will be assessed. Prospective professionals will learn what is tested (p 183). In teacher-education programmes Woolfolk (p 183) notes the work of researchers who indicate that 'testing for content mastery works against programmic goals of reflection and inquiry'.

Reed and Procter (1993) have tackled this difficult question by pointing to the lock-step situation nursing programmes are in as they meet the criteria of higher education for assessment of formal knowledge without comparative concerns for practical knowledge. The debate centres on the assessment of students' achievement in the learning strategies that have evolved to embrace reflective thinking and practice, such as critical incident technique, learning diaries and clinical studies assignments. 'The assessment of such strategies, however, remains contentious and problematic' (p 164).

Reed and Procter report that the pass/fail debate in assessment of self-reflection in the above strategies emphasizes the difficulty of making an assessment judgement. Critical incident techniques are not assessed. On the other hand, the learning diaries are structured to encourage students to avoid emotional response to situations and to use academic language when reporting them. The diary is not marked as pass/fail but used as part of the formative assessment (p 168). The authors include details of the diary structure in their text.

Challenging the prevailing methodologies of assessing clinical performance in relation to reflective practice Reed and Procter (1993, p 179) suggest the development of a method which 'is interactive and integrated, one which studies both thought and action'. This method would lead away from the right/wrong dichotomy of practice towards a valid/invalid system to take into consideration the situation in which the action took place and to allow the reasoning of the practitioner to be included. Dialogue between the assessor and the assessee follows as a necessary component of assessment, although, as the authors note, this is not without many problems. Assessing reflective practice remains an open and significant question for nurse education undergraduate programmes.

There is support for the concept of an integrated and interactive assessment of clinical practice from the work of the Australian Nursing Council Incorporated (ANCI) in the development of competencies, including reflective practice, for assessment of registration nurses. 'Reflective practice: contains those competencies relating to self-appraisal, professional development of self and others and the value of research. Reflection in practice, feelings and beliefs and the consequences of these for clients was considered an important professional benchmark' (Australian Nursing Council, 1994, p 7).

Although reflective practice is one of five major domains, it is clear that the philosophy of reflective practice has had a strong influence in the selection of the method of assessment. There is a holistic and contextual emphasis in the method. This enables opportunities of interaction between assessor and assessee, integration of context with practical action and allowance of recognition of the reasoning underlying the action of the assessee.

There are four elements in the assessment process:

- self-assessment by the nurse;
- observations by the assessor;
- interviews by the assessor with the nurse and appropriate others;
- analysis by the assessor of all relevant documentation (p 17).

Departing from a written assessment tool, the assessor uses the competency standards as a reference and pen and paper for recording her/his observations. 'The nurse assessor is the assessment tool' (Australian Nursing Council, 1994, p 13).

IMPROVING THE RELIABILITY OF CLINICAL PERFORMANCE ASSESSMENT

All these methods of assessing clinical performance experience problems in reliability derived from the fact that the examiner is required to make a judgement about the student's performance. Clinical examiners may differ in the standards they set; a single student may receive two quite different marks from two different examiners who are using different criteria to judge competence. Thus observation of performance may not be a reliable way to assign marks or grades unless preventive measures are taken.

ACTIVITY

Suggest ways in which the reliability of assessment of clinical performance can be improved.

FEEDBACK

This question has exercised the minds of nurse educators more than any other issue in assessment. Basically, reliability can be improved by achieving consensus on specific unambiguous criteria, by making those criteria known to examiners, by incorporating the criteria into assessment tools, by testing and training examiners to use those tools, by basing assessments on a sample of student behaviour rather than a single episode and by checking on the statistical profile of assessment marks.

Consensus on criteria can only be achieved by involving assessors or examiners in the development of learning objectives and assessment tools. Pre-assessment conferences can be used to achieve consensus where necessary, to discuss criteria with new teachers or assessors and to train assessors in the use of the assessment tools. After the assessments have been completed, statistical profiles of student performance and examiner performance can be used to identify atypical or isolated performance difficulties of students and characteristic marking behaviours of assessors (some mark consistently high and some consistently low). Armed with this information you can make more reliable judgements about overall student performance, you can alter the weight given to certain assessments and you can plan future teams of assessors who balance each other or may be able to influence each other to more closely approach the norm of marking practice.

CHARACTERISTICS OF A GOOD ASSESSMENT

Deciding on the purposes of assessment and the types of assessment most suited to the learning objectives is only part of the assessment task. Making your chosen assessment methods good ones is also very important.

What is a good assessment?

ACTIVITY

Based on your experience and what you have read in this chapter so far list the characteristics of a good assessment.

FEEDBACK

A good assessment is valid

An assessment is said to be valid if it tests what it is supposed to test. Assessments should test important skills, knowledge and attitudes that are the objectives of the course.

For example, an essay test used to assess a student's ability to perform a procedure is not a valid test. It tests only what the student knows should be done, but does not test whether the student is actually able to do it. A valid test of this skill would be the actual performance, under real or simulated conditions, of the procedure.

A good assessment is comprehensive

The assessment should test achievement of the essential objectives of the course and a wide and representative range of the other objectives of the course. Many assessments test only the student's memory for facts. A good test will require students to apply facts to the solution of problems or the discussion of important issues, or the performance of manual skills. Higher-level objectives should be adequately represented among assessment criteria. This means that a variety of assessment methods must be used.

A good assessment is fair

All students must have an equal chance to perform well if they have learned well. Examination items should be specific and unambiguous so that there is no risk that some students might give a wrong answer because they have mistaken the meaning of the question. If possible, tests should be spread over a period of time so that students who are having an 'off day' for some reason or another have an opportunity to be assessed under more favourable circumstances. In assessments of clinical performance, steps should be taken to provide for a variety of assessments and assessors to avoid errors due to bias of observers or other extraneous factors.

Marking schemes for questions such as MCQs should be developed so that students who know the right answer score more, on average, than students who are just guessing.

A good assessment is reliable

You must be able to rely on the consistency and accuracy of scores given. Reliability of assessors can be tested by asking two different examiners to assess the same student on achievement of the same objectives, or by asking the same examiner to assess the same test at two different times. If the scores are similar or the same then the assessment is reliable. Loustau *et al.* (1980), using videotapes to establish rater reliability for assessing clinical performance, found that cognitive items were more difficult to reach agreement on than skill items. Training sessions using videotaped student–patient interactions improved the reliability of raters using a clinical evaluation tool.

Assessments using MCQs and MEQs are very reliable because there is one agreed answer and examiners do not have to exercise judgement in giving scores. MCQs are frequently marked by computers. Unfortunately, while these exams are very reliable they are not valid for a wide range of objectives in nursing.

Essay questions, oral examinations, examination of student products such as assignments, nursing reports and projects, and direct observation of clinical performance, while being more valid assessments of nursing objectives, are frequently not very reliable because they require examiners to exercise their judgement and opinions about student performance. Reliability of these types of assessment can be improved by:

- training examiners in the application of standard criteria to establish inter-rater reliability;
- providing standard checklists or rating scales which make criteria explicit;
- averaging the scores given by more than one examiner.

A good assessment is economical

Assessments should be economical in time as well as money. Essays are very time-consuming to mark but do not take long to set whereas MCQs are quick to mark but their development is time-consuming. Clinical observation schedules that are lengthy and not feasible within normal ward routines have very little chance either of being used as they are intended or of providing valid and reliable results.

A good assessment can be used to help students learn. Assessments should, wherever possible, be a learning experience for students. In informal assessment, students can be encouraged to develop skills in peer- and self-assessment. In formal assessment for certification or mastery, students should be informed of criteria used to make judgements and of their personal performance in relation to those criteria. Formative assessment should be an integral part of learning and students should always have access to an adviser with whom they can discuss their achievements and their deficiencies.

A good assessment can give you information about the success of your course.

Assessments should be regarded by you as a research tool to help you identify patterns in your students' performance that may indicate problems with curriculum, prerequisites, and objectives and implementation of your course.

SUMMARY

Students learn what they need to learn in order to pass exams. This is a fact of life. Assessments must therefore test what students must learn in order to be competent nurses. You will not be able to measure or assess all levels of learning if you use only one or a few types of assessment method. A variety of assessment methods will help you to assess a broader range of the knowledge, skills and attitudes that your students must demonstrate in order to be competent nurses.

If the assessment results are unsatisfactory, or the pass rate is low, or if significant numbers of students are not achieving mastery in a reasonable time, use the assessment results as a guide to problem areas in your course. Assessment should be a tool for improving both teaching and learning.

Evaluating teaching 9

INTRODUCTION

Since nursing, as a discipline, has become a recognized study in higher education in most countries, the evaluation of teachers of nursing in academia has become a complex activity. 'Being an academic, means, of course, constantly being exposed to scrutiny by peers within the institution and the wider international scholarly community, by students and the public alike, indeed to being constantly evaluated' (Moses, 1988, p 28). Issues of promotion and tenure as well as a evaluation of staff members' general competence occupy the time and thought of nursing teachers as they become accustomed to a system which demands a different kind of accountability than many were used to in, for example, a hospital school of nursing.

One of the components of the role of nurse teachers in higher education that is not often recognized is their contribution to curriculum design and development. This is a continuing involvement and, while you may not be a curriculum development officer, as a teacher in both classroom and clinical nursing you are in touch with the advantages and disadvantages of curriculum design, the implementation programme and course materials.

So, just as assessment of student performance is a necessary component of helping students learn to be better nurses, so assessment of teaching is a necessary component of helping you and your teaching colleagues to offer better courses (Rotem and Abbatt, 1982).

When you have completed this chapter you should be able to plan a programme of evaluation to assist you in improving the courses that you offer.

CRITERIA FOR EVALUATION

ACTIVITY

Consider the course that you teach. After working through this book you have decided to try some new approaches to that course but you would like to be able to determine whether they are effective. What criteria will you use to evaluate your new course?

FEEDBACK

Possibly the first criterion you chose to evaluate the success of your new course was students' performance in the examinations. This is as far as many teachers go in trying to determine the value of their course, but this is not far enough. You cannot be sure that student performance is totally dependent on your teaching or your course. Many other factors are also involved. For example, students may already have known a great deal of what you thought you were teaching them or they may not have performed well because they did not have sufficient background knowledge to benefit fully from your course. Or perhaps your course is taught at the same time as another more demanding course which takes most of the students' study efforts, or perhaps your students are so highly motivated that they will perform well regardless of the quality of the course you offer. For all these reasons, and more, student examination performance is only one of many criteria you could use in evaluating your course.

Table 9.1 is a summary of the criteria you might use to evaluate courses.

Table 9.1 Criteria for course evaluation

General criteria	Specific criteria
Effectiveness	Achievement of course objectives
	Retention of learning to be used in subsequent courses
	On-the-job performance
	Occurrence of unexpected outcomes (good or bad)
Acceptability	Appropriateness of objectives
	Satisfaction with resources and teaching methods
	Learning environment and climate
	Appropriateness of assessment methods

Feasibility	Time spent in course preparation
	Class hours and private study time required by students
	Ease of availability of resources
	Cost of resources (time or money)
	Availability of appropriate facilities
	Inter-relatedness with other courses – is there
	interference with timetables, assignments, exams, etc?

Of course, it may not be possible or even appropriate to use all of these criteria but they are included here to give you some idea of the options from which you can choose.

CHOICE OF CRITERIA

ACTIVITY

How would you choose which criteria to include in your evaluation?

FEEDBACK

The answer to this question depends entirely on your circumstances and the reasons why you have chosen to evaluate. For example, if budgetary restrictions are a problem for you, you may place a high priority on evaluating resources and teaching methods to determine whether expenditure is cost-effective. If, on the other hand, you have indications that students have not been performing satisfactorily in certain areas of subsequent courses you may choose to evaluate achievement of course objectives or even the appropriateness of those objectives. The rule of thumb is to begin your evaluation in an area in which either a problem has been identified or a decision has to be made (with regard to use of resources, for example).

SOURCES OF INFORMATION

Choosing criteria is only part of the problem – once you have decided where you wish to start you must then decide how you will collect information to help you make decisions about those criteria.

ACTIVITY

Refer to the list of criteria in the feedback to the first activity in this chapter and construct a table that indicates sources of information for each criterion.

FEEDBACK

Your table might look something like Table 9.2.

Table 9.2   Sources of information for evaluation criteria

Specific criteria	Sources of information
Achievement of objectives	Pre- and post-test student performance
Retention of learning	Feedback from teachers of other courses
On-the-job performance	Direct observation. Feedback from clinical supervisors. Feedback from patients. Feedback from recent graduates on their preparation for the job
Unexpected outcomes	Observations of classroom process. Interview with students
Appropriateness of objectives	'Expert opinion'. Feedback from other teachers. Information about on-the-job performance
Resources and teaching methods	Teacher opinion based on observations in class. Student opinion (questionnaire or discussion). Peer observation
Learning environment and climate	Teacher opinion. Student opinion. Peer observation
Appropriateness of assessment	Review of assessment to ensure that it reflects objectives. Profile and analysis of student performance
Time spent in course preparation	Teacher's observations
Class hours and study time	Student diaries
Availability of resources	Teacher's observations. Student feedback
Cost of resources	Teacher's observations. Administrative records
Availability of facilities	Teacher's observations. Student feedback
Inter-relatedness with other courses	Feedback from and negotiation with other teachers

If you have had to prepare a submission or application for tenure or promotion you may have questioned the validity of some of the requirements for academic advancement. While appropriate for most university disciplines, the criteria may not appear to take into consideration the weighting of clinical teaching or clinical competence in terms of the preparation and teaching time necessary.

ACTIVITY

Imagine you have been asked by your Head of School to design an evaluation programme for the school which would meet university requirements and would be appropriate for the nursing teacher's role in the nursing course, the nursing profession and academia.

FEEDBACK

No doubt you would have sought ideas and suggestions as well as support from your colleagues, as evaluation is a common concern and rarely depends on individual choice or opinion. After listing the activities of the nurse teacher's role and categorizing the result under appropriate headings, you may have reached the same conclusions as Ketefian (1977). These are: classroom teaching, advising and supporting students, clinical competence, clinical teaching, course materials, scholarship, service to university, professional contributions, service to the community.

Now try to make a grid with those categories across the page and down the left-hand side make a list of all those who could evaluate your performance in each of the categories (Table 9.3). This is certainly an exercise needing the advice of colleagues who have had, or are having, a similar teaching experience to your own. Ketefian is helpful here, as she has provided a table and indicates who would be appropriate evaluators for each category of your role.

Next, mark on the grid who you consider could evaluate each of the categories. For example, you probably considered that students could evaluate classroom teaching, clinical teaching, student support services and clinical competence. On the other hand, you probably marked yourself in all the categories across the page. The grid is useful in deciding, for each category, who best could evaluate so that you have a comprehensive view of your course. When you have completed filling in the grid, look down each vertical line and take a category – 'course material', for example. You may have marked the nursing faculty, members of faculty in other disciplines, external reviewers, administrators and yourself as appropriate evaluators. Of course, when you complete the grid for your own teaching, you are thinking of your own personal reference, which does not imply that each category must be evaluated formally.

When such a grid is submitted to a Head of School for consideration by the whole staff, the grid could be completed through discussion with staff members and could become the school's programme of staff evaluation.

You can see that a comprehensive evaluation involves collection of information from a variety of sources. It may not be appropriate or feasible to gather information from all or even most of them but the following guidelines will assist you in deciding how you wish to use some of the most important sources of feedback on your course.

STUDENT PERFORMANCE

Student performance is an important source of information for course evaluation, although, as we mentioned earlier, it is not necessarily the most important source since it provides only part of the information you

Table 9.3 Evaluation of nurse educators (Source: adapted from Ketefian, 1977)

	Classroom teaching	Clinical teaching	Clinical competence	Student services	Course materials	Scholarship	Service to university	Professional contributions	Service to community
Students									
Nursing faculty colleagues									
Faculty colleagues in other disciplines									
External reviewers									
Clinical agency staff									
Administration									
Self									

need to have. Deficiencies in student performance can indicate that there is a problem; they might even indicate in which component of the course the problem lies; but they will rarely be able to tell you exactly what is the cause of the problem. Failure to achieve some of the course objectives will be revealed on item analysis of a well constructed assessment, but you will need to use other sources of information to determine whether the students failed to achieve the objectives because they lacked relevant prerequisite learning, whether the teaching in that area was insufficient or ineffective, whether the resources were appropriate, whether there was some extraneous variable affecting student learning at the time or whether the assessment actually reflected the objectives.

An interesting study has investigated the relationship between clinical teachers' effectiveness and student performance outcomes (Krichbaum, 1994). Improvements in students' clinical performance were strongly correlated with 'the preceptors "use of objectives" in planning student learning activities, his or her "ability to ask an appropriate number of questions in a non-threatening manner", to "convey concern for the learner", to "provide an appropriate amount of feedback in a non-threatening way", and to "provide an appropriate quantity of explanation"' (p 313).

TEACHERS' OBSERVATIONS

You will notice that you, as the teacher, are an important source of information for evaluating the course. You will be aware, every time you teach, of aspects of your classes which were particularly successful and aspects which you would do differently next time. Day-to-day experiences with colleagues often gives informal feedback about teaching that may confirm your own view of your teaching performance and build self-confidence. Your colleagues may also provide useful comments on what worked for them and what did not, which gives opportunities for you to compare your attempts at similar teaching strategies. Course evaluation by direct observation requires that you take note of these experiences and use them to improve your subsequent teaching.

Moses (1988) notes that informal self-appraisal of classroom teaching often leads into more formal, self-initiated evaluation.

SELF-AUDIT

You may be concerned about a particular area of your classroom or clinical teaching, e.g. asking questions requiring students to use skills of analysis, synthesis or evaluation rather than merely recall of factual material. You could design a 'custom-made' checklist yourself (or get a colleague to assist) or you could modify a ready-made published questionnaire. This could involve you in responding to a Likert-type scale where you rate your progress (Wealthall, Edwards and Price, 1992). Self-evaluation can provide information not accessible to others but it is an interpretation of one's own merit (Moses, 1988) and is regarded as complementary to other methods of evaluation. Peer review is a more helpful method (see below) but, used for preparation for an external review of your teaching, a self-audit could offer opportunities of rehearsal.

STUDENT OPINION

Students are also an important source of information for course evaluation. Teachers sometimes object to asking for feedback from students because they fear that students are not qualified to judge or that they will be unfair in their criticism. However, Moses (1988, p 62) reports that 'there is now wide consensus that students are the most reliable judges of tertiary teachers' classroom performance'. Eley and Thomson (1992) report that, although there have been very many claims that student evaluations are biased and thus invalid and questionnaire results are unreliable, reviews of the literature 'typically conclude that with appropriately designed questionnaires and procedures, student evaluations yield valid and reliable information on teaching effectiveness, and are a viable source of such information' (p 3). A research study was conducted at Monash University (Eley and Thomson, 1992) to design and trial questionnaires covering the range of teaching activities in the university together with the design and trialling of the software to be used. The resulting system of student evaluation of teaching (MON QUE ST) includes questionnaires for evaluation of clinical teaching in medicine and nursing.

Medicine has three categories of clinical teaching:

- the clinical teacher as a role model;
- the demonstration of clinical techniques;
- students' practice of clinical techniques.

Interestingly, but not surprisingly, the nursing faculty produced a questionnaire with four categories of clinical teaching that differ from those of medicine. Only the first category is similar: the clinical teacher as a role model. The remaining categories are:

- the demonstration and explanation of nursing care;
- students' practice of nursing care;

- the support and guidance of students.

Each category has elements that require the students' response. There are 35 elements in the nursing questionnaire; for example, in the category 'students' practice of nursing care' the element includes 'as my competence improved, the clinical teacher's supervision of my activities allowed me increasing responsibility'.

Throughout the entire questionnaire, for the evaluation of lecturing, tutoring, practical class teaching, assessment of students, consultation with students and project or thesis supervision, the students' response is guided by the following direction:

The description is true for:

- all or almost all of the relevant teaching episodes;
- most of the episodes;
- about half of the episodes;
- only some of the episodes;
- very few or none of the relevant teaching episodes.

The experience of teachers who do use student feedback as a source of information is that students, when offered some responsibility, are happy to take a responsible approach. It is also important, however, to demonstrate that student feedback has been considered and, where appropriate, used for course revision, otherwise students quickly become cynical and rightly so. It is important to ask student opinion only in areas in which you are prepared to accept their judgement. For example, students might not be competent to judge whether you have presented your subject matter accurately but they are competent to judge whether you have presented it clearly or whether the resources you have recommended helped their understanding.

For some purposes, where the class is large or where you feel anonymous feedback will more accurately reflect student opinion, you may choose to use a student opinion questionnaire. For other purposes it may be more appropriate to talk personally with students individually or as a class to gain feedback on general or specific aspects of their experiences in your classes and other components of the course. The personal approach is appropriate in situations where a personal relationship already exists, as between student and clinical supervisor, and is particularly useful for maximizing the value of individual student experiences since it allows a two-way interaction and the opportunity for clarification of specific problems.

If circumstances call for a questionnaire the same principles apply as to any form of questionnaire design – decide what information you want, determine whether a free response or rating scale would give you the most useful information, write the questions and pilot test the instrument before administering it to the students. Useful advice on the development of instruments for student evaluation of teaching can be found in Centra (1980, 1987) and Eley and Thomson (1992.)

Remember that you may be teaching registered nurses in postgraduate courses. Their considered opinion after some experience of professional and clinical work could offer valuable feedback on your teaching and on your course.

Student opinion is probably most appropriately sought in a context in which it provides private feedback to the teacher concerned. Use of student feedback for administrative decision-making such as promotion is a sensitive area and one which should be fully explored and discussed with teachers to ensure its appropriate and effective use without destruction of morale.

PEER OBSERVATION

Another major source of information is your teaching colleagues – or, if your school has an educational development unit, you may wish to ask the staff of that unit to provide a professional appraisal of your course design, your resources or your teaching performance.

Brown and Ward-Griffin (1994) have reviewed the use of peer evaluation in promoting nursing faculty effectiveness. They offer five recommendations as criteria for effective peer evaluation. In brief, the recommendations are as follows.

- The overall faculty evaluation approach must be developed by the faculty with administrative support.
- Peer evaluation should be only one component of the faculty evaluation system and the main purpose of peer evaluation is the improvement of teaching and learning.
- Peer evaluation is threatening: considerable effort needs to be made to ensure a systematic and equitable process.
- Observers need to be trained; repeated and multiple observations are recommended; measures need to be simple reliable and valid and feedback needs to be constructive, with follow-up faculty development programmes.
- In circumstances where peer evaluation meets criteria of sound evaluation measures, the results may be used for summative evaluation purposes.

(Source: adapted from Brown and Ward-Griffin, 1994, p 304)

Understandably, many teachers have no wish to expose their weaknesses to their colleagues and many opportunities are therefore missed for teachers to help each other to improve the courses they teach. This state of affairs has not been helped by the practice, in some schools, of conducting formal evaluations of teaching for administrative purposes, such as salary grading or promotion. A purely administrative approach to teacher evaluation can be counterproductive because, although it rewards teaching accomplishments, it tends to generate a climate of threat, which is not conducive to development of teaching skills for personal satisfaction or for the benefit of the students. Evaluation of teaching which emphasizes personal development and job satisfaction rather than administrative rewards should generate a more positive learning environment within the school. An approach that stresses mutual co-operation among teachers will be more helpful than one in which teachers are encouraged to criticize each other's efforts.

Discussing course changes and plans and eliciting comments from other teachers helps an atmosphere of openness to develop. This is particularly relevant if your course is likely to affect students' study habits and therefore spill over into other courses. For example, adoption of a mastery-based approach will have implications for timetabling in other courses to avoid clashes of assessment periods; checking whether this has happened and whether problems or benefits have been created for other teachers should be part of your course evaluation. Remember, your courses do not occur in isolation and therefore should not be evaluated in isolation but in the context of their relationship to other courses and the overall objectives of the programme. Anatomy classes must prepare students for what they will need to do in safely administering intramuscular injections. If they do not, then they are not effective, no matter how well the students have performed in the anatomy examination.

OBSERVATION OF CLINICAL TEACHING

As we noted in Monash University's project on student evaluation of teaching (above), clinical teaching was included and a questionnaire was designed to meet the special requirements of teaching students in a clinical setting. As clinical teachers know, planning and preparation with students and with the clinical agency staff, and the selection of clinical placements and assignments, are all part of the clinical teacher's task. The quality of the learning environment is influential in determining whether the clinical experience is positive or negative for students and, in turn, reflects on the quality of the course as a whole. Briefing and debriefing sessions assist students to clarify their expectations and to learn from the experience. A comprehensive observation of clinical teaching takes in all aspects and the information derived from a thorough review provides essential material for course evaluation (Zimmerman and Westfall, 1988).

CLINICAL COMPETENCE

Valiga and Streubert (1991) raise the issue of whether nurse teachers can be expected to be clinical experts in addition to their primary role as teachers, rather than practitioners. However, they agree with Stafford and Graves (1978) that 'students need teachers who can function well as role models, thereby demonstrating the skills, attitudes and values that all students hope to develop'. Given that students often say that clinical experience is their most potent source of learning, it follows that the clinical teacher's clinical credibility is an important component of the role (Fawcett and McQueen, 1994). In a study by Wiseman (1994), students identified 28 role-model behaviours teachers practised in the clinical setting, affirming that clinical teachers are considered role models by their students. Wiseman suggests that the specific role-model behaviours identified in the study could be used in the evaluation of both students and clinical teachers.

PERUSAL OF COURSE MATERIALS

Evaluation of teaching extends to the course and teaching materials you choose for particular topics and students. Ideally, the materials should reflect the programme's goals and conceptual framework. Selecting materials appropriate to the level of students means identifying materials that challenge and extend students rather than those that present the *status quo*. Included in the review of course documents would be course objectives and content, teaching/learning strategies, selection of clinical placements and clinical assignments, and assessment and examination methods. Review of materials can act as a valuable source of information about how closely the course adheres to the original philosophy and conceptual framework.

GUIDANCE AND SUPPORT OF STUDENTS

The extent to which you are able to identify the individual needs of your students for remedial work, helpful references and individual study plans, and offer guidance on personal problems (when asked), is a reflection of your accessibility to students (Valiga and Streubert, 1991). A successful course is often dependent on the insight of staff to identify specific learning problems and to acknowledge the achievements of successful students.

MUTUAL DEBRIEFING SESSIONS

Wealthall, Edwards and Price (1992) suggest that the teacher and students should, before a teaching session, negotiate a certain amount of time and space to debrief to each other after the session. A debriefing structure could be agreed, such as:

- 'Please continue to . . .'
- 'Try not to . . .'
- 'Why don't you . . .'

and so on.

As debriefing usually occurs as soon as possible after a teaching or practice session, the comments are likely to be relevant, pertinent and constructive.

UNINTENDED OUTCOMES

Don't forget that, even though you have defined objectives and assessed your students' achievement of those objectives, and evaluated your course partially on how well students have achieved the objectives, other outcomes of learning, which were not planned, might occur. Sometimes these will be desirable outcomes and sometimes they will not be; however, if you are not alert to the possibility of unintended outcomes you will not identify them and will miss opportunities for improving your course.

REPORTING EVALUATION DATA

This chapter assumes that you are evaluating your course mainly for your own benefit and for the benefit of your students. Other reasons for evaluation would be for research purposes, to prove the superiority or cost-effectiveness of some teaching approach, or for administrative purposes to allow official decisions to be made about administrative actions such as curriculum review or teacher promotion. Consideration of both of those purposes is beyond the scope of this book, but details of evaluation for administrative decision-making can be found in Roe and

McDonald (1983) and Joint Committee on Standards for Educational Evaluation (1981).

To the extent that your course forms part of a larger educational programme, you have a responsibility to share the results of evaluation with colleagues. This is perhaps not as important in areas such as personal evaluation of teaching performance but it is very important in areas that indicate the effectiveness of particular teaching or assessment methods – the appropriateness of course objectives and the readiness of students to learn certain aspects of the course and to use certain resources and facilities. In addition, since you have probably involved colleagues and students in providing you with information and feedback, it is important that you demonstrate that their efforts were worthwhile by discussing proposed actions with them and indicating how their feedback assisted you to make the decisions you have taken.

The way you communicate the results of your evaluation efforts will depend on your particular situation: some teachers choose to publish in the professional literature to gain a wider audience. Some offer in-house seminars or establish regular review meetings of interested teachers, and some choose informal discussions over a cup of coffee. Whichever your preference, remember that feedback on teaching is most effective when it is framed constructively, when it offers specific indicators for improvement and when it is supported by concrete examples rather than abstract ideals. Don't be overly concerned if some of your information is derived from subjective opinions as these are the best indicators of learning environment, an important aspect of nursing education. 'Anthropological' approaches to evaluation have been shown to be as effective as experimental approaches in providing feedback to teachers which they are prepared to accept (Schermerhorn and Williams, 1979). In addition, observational, even anecdotal, data may be more valid in the evaluation of much of nursing education than is an attempt to experimentally prove that 'method A' is better than 'method B'. The literature abounds with such research-oriented evaluations, which are almost always confounded by the multitude of uncontrollable variables occurring in any educational programme.

Evaluation of teaching should be an ongoing part of every teacher's teaching and learning programme. Information may be sought formally or informally, verbally or through questionnaires or course documents, or it may be collected along the way as critical incidents or unexpected outcomes make themselves apparent. Whatever the source of the information, it should be evaluated for its potential contribution to better student learning and, where possible and desirable, changes should be implemented and evaluated in their turn.

SUMMARY

ACTIVITY

Develop a plan for conducting an evaluation of your course.

FEEDBACK

Use the following checklist to ensure that you have included the necessary steps in your course evaluation plan.

CHECKLIST FOR COURSE EVALUATION

- Why do you wish to carry out an evaluation? Is the purpose for improvement, for research or for administrative reasons?
- What questions will you ask to provide you with information suited to your purposes?
- What sources of information will you use?
- What instruments or resources will you need for the acquisition of that information?
- How will you analyse and use the data you gather?
- What are the factors in the context or climate of your school that will determine the way you report your evaluation results?
- What methods will you use for reporting the results of your evaluation that you have decided to make public?
- How will you plan to implement changes which are indicated by your evaluation? (Consider the context of your course.)
- How will you evaluate the changes you have made?

We hope that this book will have helped you both to evaluate your teaching efforts and to plan appropriate educational responses to what you learn about your programme. Teaching and learning is a dynamic process: healthy educational programmes, like children, are those that continue to develop. Your ability and willingness to adapt to changing needs and contexts will serve as a valuable model for the flexibility your students will need as professionals practising in a rapidly changing environment.

References

Abbatt, F. (1992) *Teaching for Better Learning. A Guide for Teachers of Primary Health Care Staff*, WHO, Geneva.

Abercrombie, M. (1969) *The Anatomy of Judgement*, Penguin, Harmondsworth.

Adkins, D. (1974) *Test Construction*, 2nd edn, Charles E. Merrill, Columbus, OH.

Allen, M. (1977) *Evaluation of Educational Programmes in Nursing*, WHO, Geneva.

Allmark, P. (1995) Can there be an ethics of care? *Journal of Medical Ethics*, **21**, 19–24.

Andersen, B. (1989) Problem based learning in nursing education: justified or a response to fashion? Paper presented to Education Department, School of Medicine, Southern Illinois University, Springfield, IL, November.

Andersen, B. (1990) The case for learner-managed learning in health professionals' education. Paper presented at 1st International Learner Managed Learning Conference, London, April.

Andersen, B. (1991) Mapping the terrain of the discipline, in *Towards a Discipline of Nursing*, (eds G. Gray and R. Pratt), Churchill Livingstone, Melbourne, Victoria.

Anderson, J. (1981) The MCQ controversy – a review. *Medical Teacher*, **3**, 150–156.

Andersen, S. L. (1989) The nurse advocate project: a strategy to retain new graduates. *JONA*, **19**(12), 26.

Armitage, P. and Burnard, P. (1991) Mentors or preceptors? Narrowing the theory–practice gap. *Nurse Education Today*, **11**, 225–229.

Aroskar, M. (1980) Anatomy of an ethical dilemma. *American Journal of Nursing*, **80**, 658–663.

Australian Nursing Council (1994) *Using the ANCI Competencies. An Assessment Kit*, Australian Nursing Council Incorporated, Canberra.

Ausubel, D. (1960) The use of advance organisers in the learning and retention of meaningful verbal material. *Journal of Educational Psychology*, **51**, 267–272.

Baldwin, D. and Price, S. (1994) Work excitement. The energiser for home health care nursing. *JONA*, **24**(9), 37–42.

Ball, M. J., Hannah, K., Jelger, U. and Petersen, H (eds) (1988) *Nursing Informatics. Where Caring and Technology Meet*, Springer, New York.

Barrows, H. and Tamblyn, R. (1980) *Problem-based Learning. An Approach to Medical Education*, Springer, New York.

Battenfield, B. (1986) *Designing Clinical Evaluation Tools: The State of the Art*, National League for Nursing, New York.

Beare, H. and Slaughter, R. (1993) *Education for the Twenty-first Century*, Routledge, London.

Beddome, G., Budgen, C., Hills, M. *et al.* (1995) Education and practice collaboration: a strategy for curriculum development. *Journal of Nursing Education*, 34(1), 11–15.

Benner, P. (1982) From novice to expert. *American Journal of Nursing*, **Mar**, 402–407.

Benner, P. (1984) *From Novice to Expert: Excellence and Power in Clinical Practice*, Addison-Wesley, Menlo Park, CA.

Benner, P. (1989) Performance expectations of new graduates. Unpublished paper, AACN Invitational Conference. Critical Care Nursing at the Baccalaureate Level. Strategies for the Future, University of California, San Francisco School of Nursing.

Bennett, J. and Kingham, M. (1993) Learning diaries, in *Nurse Education. A Reflective Approach*, (eds J. Reed and S. Procter), Edward Arnold, Sevenoaks.

Benoliel, J. (1983) Ethics in nursing practice and education. *Nursing Outlook*, 31, 211–215.

Bernal, E. and Bush, E. (1985) Values clarification: a critique. *Journal of Nursing Education*, 24(4), 174–175.

Bersky, A. and Yocom, C. (1994) Computerised clinical simulation testing. Its use for competence assessment in nursing. *Nursing and Health Care*, 15(3), 120–127.

Bevis, E. (1982) *Curriculum Building in Nursing: A Process*, C. V. Mosby, St Louis, MO.

Bevis, E. (1989) The curriculum consequences: aftermath of revolution, in *Curriculum Revolution: Reconceptualizing Nursing Education*, National League for Nursing Publication No. 15-2280, National League for Nursing, New York.

Bevis, E. and Watson, J. (1989) *Toward a Caring Curriculum: A New Pedagogy for Nursing*, National League for Nursing Publication No. 15-2278, National League for Nursing, New York.

Biggs, J. (1989) Approaches to the enhancement of tertiary teaching. *Higher Education Research and Development*, 8(1), 7–25.

Biggs, J. and Telfer, R. (1983) *The Process of Learning*, Prentice-Hall, Collingwood, Victoria.

Biscoe, G. (1989) The future: planning, reformation, uncertainty, in *Issues in Australian Nursing 2*, (eds G. Gray and R. Pratt), Churchill Livingstone, Melbourne, Victoria.

Bligh, D. (1972) *What's the Use of Lectures?* Penguin, Harmondsworth.

Block, J. (1971) Introduction to mastery learning; theory and practice, in *Mastery Learning: Theory and Practice*, (ed. J. Block), Holt, Rinehart & Winston, New York.

Bloom, B. (1971) Mastery learning, in *Mastery Learning: Theory and Practice*, (ed. J. Block), Holt, Rinehart & Winston, New York.

Bondy, K. N. (1983) Criterion-referenced definitions for rating scales in clinical education. *Journal of Nursing Education*, 22, 376–382.

Boud, D. (1988) How to help students learn from experience, in *The Medical Teacher*, (eds K. Cox and C. Ewan), Churchill Livingstone, Edinburgh.

Boud, D. and Feletti, G. (eds) (1991) *The Challenge of Problem Based Learning*, Kogan Page, London.

Boud, D., Keogh, R. and Walker, D. (1985) *Reflection: Turning Experience into Learning*, Kogan Page, London.

Brady, L. (1992) *Curriculum Development*, Prentice-Hall, Brunswick, Victoria.

Brookfield S. (1989) *Developing Critical Thinkers*, Jossey Bass, San Francisco, CA.

Brookfield S. (1991) *The Skillful Teacher. On Technique, Trust and Responsiveness in the Classroom*, Jossey-Bass, San Francisco, CA.

Brown, B. and Ward-Griffin, C. (1994) The use of peer evaluation in promoting nursing faculty teaching effectiveness: a review of the literature. *Nurse Education Today*, **14**, 299–305.

Brown, G. (1978) *Lecturing and Explaining*, Methuen, London.

Bruner, J. (1962) *On Knowing*, Harvard University Press, Cambridge, MA.

Bruner, J., Goodnow, J. and Austin, G. (1956) *A Study of Thinking*, John Wiley & Sons, New York.

Burnard, P. (1987) Towards an epistemological basis for experiential learning in nurse education. *Journal of Advanced Education*, **12**, 189–193.

Burrows, M. (1993) Strategies for staff development. *Canadian Nurse*, **89**(2), 32–34.

Carpenito, L. and Duespohl, T. (1985) *A Guide for Effective Clinical Instruction*, 2nd edn, Aspen, Rockville.

Carr, W. and Kemmis, S. (1986) *Becoming Critical: Knowing Through Action Research*, Deacon University Press, Geelong, Victoria.

Casbergue, J. (1978) Role of faculty development in clinical education (Appendix 14A), in *Evaluating Clinical Competence in the Health Professions*, (eds M. Morgan and D. Irby), C. V. Mosby, St Louis, MO, pp 185–186.

Centra, J. (1980) *Determining Faculty Effectiveness*, Jossey-Bass, San Francisco, CA.

Centra, J. (1987) Formative and summative evaluation: parody or paradox? *New Directions for Teaching and Learning*, **30**, 47–55.

Clark, C. (1987) *The Nurse as Group Leader*, 2nd edn, Springer, New York.

Clay, T. (1992) Education and empowerment: securing nursing's future. *International Nursing Review*, **39**(1), 15–17.

Conley, V. (1973) *Curriculum and Instruction in Nursing*, Little, Brown, Boston, MA.

Coombs, E., Jabbusch, B., Jones, M. *et al.* (1981) An incremental approach to self-directed learning. *Journal of Nursing Education*, **20**, 30–35.

Corey, G., Corey, M. and Callanan, P. (1993) *Issues and Ethics in the Helping Professions*, 4th edn, Brooks/Cole, Pacific Grove, CA.

Cottier, L. (1986) *Nurse Education and Australian Studies*. Project Report. CRASTE Paper No. 14, December.

Cottrell, B., Cox, B., Kelsey, S. *et al.* (1986) A clinical evaluation tool for nursing students based on the nursing process. *Journal of Nursing Education*, **25**(7), 270–274.

Cox, H., Hanna, B. and Peart, K. (1994) *The Joint Appointment*, in *Unifying Nursing Practice and Theory*, (eds J. Lathlean and B. Vaughan), Butterworth Heinemann, Oxford.

Cox, H., Harsanyi, B. and Dean, L. C. (1987) *Computers and Nursing. Application to Practice, Education and Research*, Appleton & Lange, Norwalk, CT.

Cox, K. (1987) Knowledge which cannot be used is useless. *Medical Teacher*, 9(2), 145–154.

Crittenden, B. (1994) Higher Education Supplement, *The Australian*, **Sep 14**, 29.

Cronbach, L. and Snow, R. (1977) *Aptitudes and Instructional Methods*, Irvington, New York.

Crotty, M. (1989) Using an alternative model to design a Registered General Nurse curriculum. *Nurse Education Today*, 9, 46–52.

Curtin, L (1978) A proposed model for critical analysis. *Nursing Forum*, 17, 12–17.

Dachelet, C., Wemett, M., Garling, E. *et al.* (1981) The critical incident technique applied to the evaluation of the clinical practicum setting. *Journal of Nursing Education*, 20, 15–31.

Davis, A. (1979) Ethics rounds with intensive care nurses. *Nursing Clinics of North America*, 14, 45–55.

Davis, A. and Aroskar, M. (1978) *Ethical Dilemmas and Nursing Practice*, Appleton-Century-Crofts, New York.

Davis, A. and Krueger, J. (eds) (1980) *Patients, Nurses and Ethics*, American Journal of Nursing Co., New York.

D'Cruz, J. V. and Tham, G. N. (1993) *Nursing and Nursing Education in Multicultural Australia. A Victorian Study of Some Cultural Curriculum and Demographic Issues*, David Lovell Publishing, Melbourne, Victoria.

Dewey, J. (1917) *Democracy and Education*, Macmillan, New York.

Dewey, J. (1938) *Experience and Education*, Macmillan, New York.

Donaldson, S. and Crowley, D. (1978) The discipline of nursing. *Nursing Outlook*, 26, 113–120.

Dressel, P. (1980) *Improving Degree Programs*, Jossey-Bass, San Francisco, CA.

Dunn, D. (1986) Assessing the development of clinical nursing skills. *Nurse Education Today*, 6, 28–35.

Eason, F. R. and Corbett, R. W. (1991) Effective teacher characteristics identified by adult learners in nursing. *Journal of Continuing Education in Nursing*, 22(1), 23.

Eble, K. (1988) *The Craft of Teaching*, Jossey-Bass, San Francisco, CA.

Eley, M. and Thomson, M. (1992) *A System for Student Evaluation of Teaching*, Higher Education Advisory and Research Unit, Monash University, Melbourne, Victoria.

Emden, C. (1991) Ways of knowing in nursing, in *Towards a Discipline of Nursing*, (eds G. Gray and R. Pratt), Churchill Livingstone, Melbourne, Victoria.

Engel, C. (1980) For the use of objectives. *Medical Teacher*, 2, 232–237.

Ericksen, S. (1984) *The Essence of Good Teaching*, Jossey-Bass, San Francisco, CA.

Fahy, K. and Lumby, J. (1988) Clinical assessment in a college program. *Australian Journal of Advanced Nursing*, 5(4), 5–9.

Fawcett, J. (1989) *Analysis and Evaluation of Conceptual Models of Nursing*, F. A. Davis, Philadelphia, PA.

Fawcett, T. N. and McQueen, A. (1994) Clinical credibility and the role of the nurse teacher. *Nurse Education Today*, 14, 264–271.

Feletti, G. (1993) Inquiry based and problem based learning: how similar are these approaches to nursing and medical education? *Higher Education Research and Development*, **12**(2), 143–156.

Fenner, K. (1980) *Ethics and Law in Nursing: Professional Perspectives*, D. van Nostrand, New York.

Fishel, A. and Johnson, G. (1981) The three-way conference – nursing student, nursing supervisor and nursing educator. *Journal of Nursing Education*, **20**, 18–23.

Fivars, G. and Gosnell, D. (1966) *Nursing Evaluation: The Problem and the Process. The Critical Incident Technique*, Macmillan, New York.

Flanagan, G. (1954) The critical incident technique. *Psychological Bulletin*, **51**, 327–358.

Fothergill-Bourbonnais, F. and Higuchi, K. (1995) Selecting clinical learning experiences: an analysis of the factors involved. *Journal of Nursing Education*, **34**(1), 37–41.

Fraenkel, J. (1980) *Helping Students Think and Value Strategies for Teaching the Social Studies*, Prentice-Hall, Englewood Cliffs, NJ.

Freire, P. (1970) *Pedagogy of the Oppressed*, Seabury Press, New York.

Gagne, R. (1976) *Essentials of Learning for Instruction*, Dryden Press, Hinsdale, IL.

Garbin, M. (ed.) (1991) *Assessing Educational Outcomes*, National League for Nursing Press, New York.

Geach, B. (1974) The problem-solving technique: is it relevant to practice? *Canadian Nurse*, **Jan**, 21–22.

Gesse, T. and Dempsey, P. (1981) Debate as a teaching-learning strategy. *Nursing Outlook*, **Jul** 421–423.

Gibson, S. (1980) A critique of the objectives model of curriculum design applied to the education and training of district nurses. *Journal of Advanced Nursing*, 5, 161–167.

Gillette, J. and McCollom, M. (eds) (1990) *Small Groups in Context*, Addison-Wesley, Menlo Park, CA.

Girod, G. (1973) *Writing and Assessing Attitudinal Objectives*, Charles E. Merrill, Columbus, OH.

Gonczi, A., Haager, P. and Oliver, L. (1990) *Establishing Competency-Based Standards in the Professions*. Research Paper No. 1 NOOSR, Australian Government Printing Service, Canberra.

Goodall, H. (1990) *Small Group Communications in Organizations*, Brown Publishers, Dubuque, IA.

Gordon, M. (1978) Assessment of student affect: a clinical approach, in *Evaluating Clinical Competence in the Health Professions*, (eds M. Morgan and D. Irby), C. V. Mosby, St Louis, MO.

Gray, G. and Pratt, R. (eds) (1991) *Towards a Discipline of Nursing*, Churchill Livingstone, Melbourne, Victoria.

Greaves, F. (1987) *Nurse Education and the Curriculum. A Curricular Model*, Chapman & Hall, London.

Habermas, J. (1979) *Communication and the Evolution of Society*, Beacon Press, Boston, MA.

Haddad, A. and Kapp, M. (1991) *Ethical and Legal Issues in Home Health Care*, Appleton & Lange, Norwalk, CT.

Hamilton, M. (1981) Mentorhood: a key to nursing leadership. *Nursing Leadership*, **4**(1), 4–8.

Hannafin, M. J. and Peck, K. L. (1988) *The Design, Development and Evaluation of Instructional Software*, Macmillan, New York.

Heath, J. (1982) *Curriculum Design in Nursing. A Practical Guide for Course Planners*, NHS Learning Resources Unit, Sheffield.

Heath, J. and Marson, S. (1979) It's a taxing process. *Nursing Mirror*, Aug 23, 75–78.

Henderson, V. (1966) *The Nature of Nursing*, Macmillan, New York.

Henderson, V. (1991) *Reflections After 25 Years*, National League for Nursing Publication No. 15-2346, National League for Nursing, New York.

Hengstberger-Sims, C. (1987) An evaluation of nursing re-entry and employment (refresher) programs conducted by the New South Wales College of Nursing during June 1985-1986. A project submitted in partial fulfilment for the degree of Master of Health Personnel Education, University of New South Wales, Sydney, NSW.

Henry, S. and Ensunsa, K. (1991) Preceptorship in nursing service and education, in *Review of Research in Nursing Education*, vol. IV, (eds P. Baj and G. Clayton), National League for Nursing Publication No. 15-2376, National League for Nursing, New York, pp 51–72.

Higgins, L. (1994) Integrating background nursing experience and study at the postgraduate level: an application of problem-based learning. *Higher Education Research and Development*, **13**(1), 23–33.

Hill, B. (1991) *Values Education in Australian Schools*, Australian Council for Educational Research, Hawthorn, Victoria.

Hillegas, K. and Valentine, S. (1986) Development and evaluation of a summative clinical grading tool. *Journal of Nursing Education*, **25**(5), 218–220.

Hogston, R. (1993) From competent novice to competent expert: a discussion of competence in the light of the post registration and practice project. *Nurse Education Today*, **13**, 167–171.

Holloway, D. and Race, A. (1993) Developing a rationale for research based practice: some considerations for nurse teachers. *Nurse Education Today*, **13**, 250–263.

Hudson, L. (1968) *Frames of Mind: Ability, Perception and Self-Perception in the Arts and Sciences*, Methuen, London.

Hunt, E. (1983) On the nature of intelligence. *Science*, **219**(4581), 141–146.

Hunt, G. (1992) What is a nursing ethics? *Nurse Education Today*, **12**(5), 323–328.

Hynes, K. (1980) An ethical system, in *Patients, Nurses and Ethics*, (eds A. Davis and J. Krueger), American Journal of Nursing Co., New York.

Illich, I. (1971) *Deschooling Society*, Harper & Row, New York.

Illich, I. (1976) *Medical Nemesis: The Expropriation of Health*, Pantheon, New York.

Illich, I. (1995) Pathogenesis, immunity and the quality of public health. *Qualitative Health Research*, **15**(1), 7–14.

Infante, M. (1985) *The Clinical Laboratory in Nursing Education*, 2nd edn, John Wiley & Sons, New York.

Infante, M., Forbes, E., Houldin, A. and Naylor, M. (1989) A clinical teaching project: examination of a clinical teaching model. *Journal of Professional Nursing*, **5**(5), 132–139.

Irby, D. and Dohner, C. (1976) Student clinical performance, in *Teaching in the Health Professions*, (eds C. Ford and M. Morgan), C. V. Mosby, St Louis, MO.

Jackson, M. (1995) Seven steps toward a better education. *Sydney Morning Herald*, **Apr 17**, 11.

Jacques, D. (1984) *Learning in Groups*, Croom Helm, London.

Johnson, D. and Johnson, R. (1974) Instructional goal structure: co-operative, competitive or individualistic? *Review of Educational Research*, **44**, 213–241.

Johnstone, M. (1994) *Bio-ethics: A Nursing Perspective*, W. B. Saunders, Sydney, NSW.

Joint Committee on Standards for Educational Evaluation (1981) *Standards for Evaluation of Educational Programs, Projects and Materials*, McGraw Hill, New York.

Jolley, M. and Allan, P. (1986) *The Curriculum in Nursing Education*, Chapman & Hall, London.

Joorabchi, B. (1981) How to construct problem-solving MCQs. *Medical Teacher*, **3**, 9–13.

Jowers, L. and Herr, K. (1990) A review of literature on mentor-protege relationships, in *Review of Research in Nursing Education*, vol. III, (eds G. Clayton and P. Baj), National League for Nursing, New York, pp 49–76.

Kagan, J. (1965) *Impulsive and Reflective Children: Significance of Conceptual Tempo in Learning in the Educational Process*, Rand McNally, Chicago, IL.

Kamenka, E. and Tay, A. (1981) *Teaching Human Rights*, Australian Government Publishing Service, Canberra.

Kasch, C. (1986) Toward a theory of nursing action: skills and competency in nurse-patient interaction. *Nursing Research*, **35**(4), 226–230.

Katz, F. and Snow, R. (1980) *Assessing Health Workers' Performance. A Manual for Training and Supervision*, Public Health Papers No. 72, WHO, Geneva.

Kemmis, S. (1985) Action research and the politics of reflection, in *Reflection: Turning Experience into Learning*, (eds D. Boud, R. Keogh and D. Walker), Routledge, London.

Kenway, J. and Watkins, P. (1994) *Nurses, Power Politics and Post-Modernity*, University of New England Press, Armidale, NSW.

Kermode, S. (1985) Clinical supervision in nurse education: some parallels with teacher education. *Australian Journal of Advanced Nursing*, **2**(3), 39–45.

Kermode, S. and Brown, C. (1995) Where have all the flowers gone? Nursing's escape from the radical critique. *Contemporary Nurse*, **4**(1), 8–15.

Kerr, F. (ed.) (1976) *Changing the Curriculum*, Unibooks, London.

Ketefian, S. (1977) A paradigm for faculty evaluation. *Nursing Outlook*, **34**(4), 188–192.

Kirby, S. (1977) Testing: for what purpose? Norm-referencing or criterion-referencing? *Lamp*, **Aug**, 27–29.

Kirby, S. (1982) *Nursing Undergraduate Review for Self Education*, AIDS Health Science Press, Follett, Chicago, IL.

Knowles, M. (1975) *Self-Directed Learning – A Guide for Learners and Teachers*, Association Press, Follett, Chicago, IL.

Knox, J. (1980) How to use modified essay questions. *Medical Teacher*, **2**, 20–24.

Kohlberg, L. (1972) The cognitive developmental approach to moral education. *Humanist*, **32**, 12–18.

Konner, M. (1993) *The Trouble with Medicine*, BBC Enterprises, London.

Kramer, M. (1974) *Reality Shock: Why Nurses Leave Nursing*, C. V. Mosby, St Louis, MO.

Kramer, M. (1985) Why does reality shock continue?, in *Current Issues in Nursing*, (eds J. McCloskey and H. Grace), Blackwell Scientific Publications, Boston, MA, pp 891–903.

Kramer, N. (1993) Preceptorship policy: a tool for success. *Journal of Continuing Education in Nursing*, **24**(6), 274–276.

Krichbaum, K. (1994) Clinical teaching effectiveness described in relation to learning outcomes of baccalaureate nursing students. *Journal of Nursing Education*, **33**(7), 306–316.

Krumme, U. S. (1975) The case for criterion-referenced measurement. *Nursing Outlook*, **23**, 764–779.

Kruse, L. and Fagerbarger, D. (1982) Development and implementation of a contract grading system. *Journal of Nursing Education*, **21**, 31–37.

Labunski, A. (1991) Behavioural competencies for nursing practice. *Nursing Outlook*, **39**(4), 174–177.

Laduca, A (1975) Professional performance situation model for health professions education: occupational therapy, as quoted in *Competency Based Curriculum Development in Medical Education: An Introduction*, (W. McGaghie, G. Miller, A. Sajid and T. Telder), WHO, Geneva.

Latchem, G., Williamson, J. and Henderson-Lancett, L. (1993) *Interactive Multimedia: Practice and Promise*, Kogan Page, London.

Lathlean, J. (1992) The contribution of lecturer practitioners to theory and practice in nursing. *Journal of Clinical Nursing*, **1**, 237–242.

Lathlean, J. and Vaughan, B. (1994) *Unifying Nursing Practice and Theory*, Butterworth Heinemann, Oxford.

Laurillard, D. (1993) *Rethinking University Thinking: A Framework for the Effective Use of Educational Technology*, Routledge, London.

Lawler, J. (1991) In search of an Australian identity, in *Towards a Discipline of Nursing*, (eds G. Gray and R. Pratt), Churchill Livingstone, Melbourne, Victoria.

Lemin, M., Potts, H. and Welsford, P. (eds) (1994) *Values Strategies for Classroom Teachers*, Australian Council for Educational Research, Hawthorn, Victoria.

Lenburg, C. and Mitchell, C. (1991) Assessment of outcomes: the design and use of real and simulation nursing performance examinations. *Nursing and Health Care*, **12**(2), 68–74.

Levine, M. E. (1988) Antecedents from adjunctive disciplines: creation of nursing theory. *Nursing Science Quarterly*, **1**, 16–21.

Lickman, P., Simms, L. and Greene, C. (1993) Learning environment: the catalyst for work excitement. *Journal of Continuing Education in Nursing*, **24**(5), 211–216.

Lindeman, C.A. (1989) Curriculum revolution: reconceptualising clinical nursing education. *Nursing and Health Care*, **Jan**, 23–28.

Lindesmith, K. and McWeeny, M. (1994) The power of storytelling. *Journal of Continuing Education in Nursing*, **25**(4) 186–187.

Loustau, A., Lentz, M., Lee, K. *et al.* (1980) Evaluating students' clinical performance: using videotape to establish rater reliability. *Journal of Nursing Education*, **19**, 10–17.

Lovell, R. (1980) *Adult Learning*, Croom Helm, London.

Lowman, J. (1984) *Mastering the Techniques of Teaching*, Jossey-Bass, San Francisco, CA.

Ludinsky, J. (1991) Reflective withdrawal through journal writing, in *Fostering Critical Reflection in Adulthood: A Guide to Transformation and Emancipatory Learning*, (eds J. Mezirow *et al.*), Jossey-Bass, San Francisco, CA.

Lumby, J. (1995) Researching the knowing through the knower. *Collegian*, **2**(1), 4–15.

Lutz, E., Elfrink, V. and Eddy, D. (1991) Research on values and values education in nursing, in *Review of Research in Nursing Education*, vol. IV, (eds P. Baj and G. Clayton), National League for Nursing Publication No. 15-2376, National League for Nursing, New York, pp 107–139.

McCauley, C. (1986) Developmental experiences in managerial work: a literature review. *Technical Report No. 26*, Centre for Creative Leadership, Greensboro, NC.

MacDonald, J. (1993) The caring imperative: a must? *Australian Journal of Advanced Nursing*, **11**(1), 26–30.

McGrath, B. and Princeton, J. (1987) Evaluation of a clinical preceptor program for new graduates – eight years later. *Journal of Continuing Education in Nursing*, **18**(4), 133–187.

McLeish, J. (1973) *The Psychology of the Learning Group*, Hutchinson, London.

MacLeod, M. and Farrell, P. (1994) The need for significant reform: a practice-driven approach to curriculum. *Journal of Nursing Education*, **33**(5), 208–214.

MacNamara, M., Meyler, M. and Arnold A. (1990) Management education and the challenge of action learning. *Higher Education*, **19**, 419–433.

Marsick, V. (ed.) (1987) *Learning in the Workplace*, Croom Helm, London.

Marsick, V. (1991) Action learning and reflection in the workplace, in *Fostering Critical Reflection in Adulthood: A Guide to Transformation and Emancipatory Learning*, (eds J. Mezirow *et al.*), Jossey-Bass, San Francisco, CA.

Martin, H. and Sheehan, J. (1985) The attitudes of nurse tutor students towards behavioural objectives: background and method of study. *Journal of Advanced Nursing*, **10**, 149–153.

Marton, F. and Saljo, R. (1984) Approaches to learning, in *The Experience of Learning*, (eds F. Marton *et al.*), Scottish Academic Press, Edinburgh.

Mascord, P. (1992) *Preceptor Guide*, The New South Wales College of Nursing, Glebe, NSW.

Maslow, A. (1943) A theory of human motivation. *Psychological Review*, **50**, 370–396.

Matheney, R. V. (1969) Pre- and post-clinical conferences for students. *American Journal of Nursing*, **69**(2), 286–289.

Matthews, R. and Veins, D. (1988) Evaluating basic nursing skills through group video testing. *Journal of Nursing Education*, **26**(1), 44–46.

Melia, K. (1982) 'Tell it as it is' – a qualitative methodology and nursing research: understanding the student's world. *Journal of Advanced Nursing*, **7**, 327–335.

Mezirow, J. (1983) A critical theory of adult learning, in *Adult Learning and Education*, (ed. M. Tight), Croom Helm, London.

Mezirow, J. (1985) A critical theory of self-directed learning, in *Self Directed Learning: From Theory to Practice*, (ed. S. Brookfield), Jossey-Bass, San Francisco, CA.

Mezirow J. et al. (1991) *Fostering Critical Reflection in Adulthood. A Guide to Transformative and Emancipatory Learning*, Jossey-Bass, San Francisco, CA.

Miles, M. (1981) *Learning to Work in Groups*, 2nd edn, Teachers' College, Columbia University, New York.

Modra, H. (1989) Using learning journals to encourage critical thinking at a distance, in *Critical Reflection in Distance Education*, (eds T. Evans and D. Nation), Taylor & Francis, Philadelphia, PA.

Morgan, B., Luke, C. and Herbert, J. (1979) Evaluating clinical proficiency. *Nursing Outlook*, **27**, 540–544.

Morgan, M. and Irby, D. (1978) *Evaluating Clinical Competence in the Health Professions*, C. V. Mosby, St Louis, MO.

Moses, I. (1988) *Academic Staff Evaluation and Development*, University of Queensland Press, St Lucia, Queensland.

Neufeld, V. and Norman, G. (eds) (1985) *Assessing Clinical Competence*, Springer, New York.

Newble, D., Dauphine, D., Dawson, B. et al. (1994) Guidelines for assessing clinical competence. *Teaching and Learning in Medicine*, **6**(3), 213–220.

Nichols, E. G., Beeken, J. E. and Wickerson, N. N. (1994) Distance delivery through compressed video. *Journal of Nursing Education*, **33**(4), 184–186.

Novak, J. and Gowin, D. (1984) *Learning How To Learn*, Cambridge University Press, New York.

Nursing Times Open Learning Programme (1991) Professional development module. *Nursing Times*, **87**(22), i–viii.

O'Brien, D. and Walton, G. (1993) An information retrieval and analysis package, in *Nurse Education. A Reflective Approach*, (eds J. Reed and S. Procter), Edward Arnold, Sevenoaks.

Oppenheim, A. (1966) *Questionnaire Design and Attitude Measurement*, Basic Books, New York.

Orton, H. (1983) Ward learning climate and student response, in *Research into Nurse Education*, (ed. B. D. Davis), Croom Helm, London.

Packer, J. L. (1994) Education for clinical practice: an alternative approach. *Journal of Nursing Education*, **33**(9), 411–416.

Parkes R. (1994) Specialization in nursing. Unpublished paper prepared on behalf of National Nursing Organizations, Canberra.

Parse, R. R. (1987) *Nursing Science: Major Paradigms, Theories and Critiques*, W. B. Saunders, Philadelphia, PA.

Pashuk, G. (1983) *Catalogue of Educational Films*, Tertiary Education Research Centre, University of New South Wales, Sydney, NSW.

Pask, G. (1976) Styles and strategies of learning. *British Journal of Educational Psychology*, **46**, 128–148.

Pederson, C., Duckett, L. and Maruyama, G. (1990) Using structured controversy to promote ethical decision making. *Journal of Nursing Education*, **29**(4), 150–157.

Penzias, A. (1989) *Ideas and Information. Managing in a High-Tech World*, W. W. Norton, New York.

Perry, A. (1991) Sociology: its contributions and critiques, in *Nursing: A Knowledge Base for Practice*, (eds A. Perry and M. Jolley) Edward Arnold, Sevenoaks.

Perry, A. and Jolley M. (eds) (1991) *Nursing: A Knowledge Base for Practice*, Edward Arnold, Sevenoaks.

Phenix, P. (1966) *Realms of Meaning*, McGraw Hill, New York.

Piaget, J. (1971) *Science of Education and the Psychology of the Child*, Longman, London.

Posner, G. J. (1985) *Field Experience. A Guide to Reflective Teaching*, Longman, New York.

Powell, L. (1973) *Lecturing*, Pitman, London.

Pratt, R. (1989) Sine qua non: the psychomotor skills profile of beginning practitioners in nursing. Unpublished masters degree major project, School of Medical Education, University of New South Wales, Sydney, NSW.

Purtilo, R. (1983) Ethics in allied health education: state of the art. *Journal of Allied Health*, **12**, 210–220.

Quinn, F. (1994) *Principles and Practice of Nurse Education*, Chapman & Hall, London.

Ramsden, P. (1988) Studying learning: improving teaching, in *Improving Learning: New Perspectives*, (ed. P. Ramsden), Kogan Page, London.

Raths, J. (1971) Teaching without specific objectives. *Educational Leadership*, 714–720.

Raths, L. (1966) *Values and Teaching*, Charles E. Merrill, Columbus, OH.

Reed, J. and Procter, S. (eds) (1993) *Nurse Education: A Reflective Approach*, Edward Arnold, Sevenoaks.

Reilly, A. (1980) *Behavioural Objectives in Evaluation in Nursing*, Appleton-Century-Crofts, New York.

Reilly, D. E. (1978) *Teaching and Evaluating the Affective Domain in Nursing Programs*, Charles B. Slack, Detroit, MI.

Reilly, D. (1989) Ethics and values in nursing: are we opening Pandora's box? *Nursing and Health Care*, **10**(2), 91–95.

Reilly, D. and Oermann, M. (1992) *The Clinical Field. Its Use in Nursing Education*, Appleton-Century Crofts, Norwalk, CT.

Revans, R. W. (1980) *Action Learning*, Blond & Briggs, London.

Riddell, R. and Wright, S. (1991) *Health Issue: Actions and Reactions*, Longman Cheshire, Melbourne, Victoria.

Rines, A. (1963) *Evaluating Student Progress in Learning the Practice of Nursing*, Teachers' College Press, Columbia University, New York.

Roe, E. and McDonald, R. (1983) *Informed Professional Judgement: A Handbook for Evaluation in Higher Education*, University of Queensland Press, St Lucia, Queensland.

Rogers, C. (1969) *Freedom to Learn*, Charles E. Merrill, Columbus, OH.

Rotem, A. and Abbatt, F. (1982) *Self-Assessment for Teachers of Health Workers*, WHO, Geneva.

Rumbold, G. (1993) *Ethics in Nursing Practice*, Baillière Tindall, London.

Ryan, G. (1989) Problem-based learning – some practical issues. *Research and Development in Higher Education*, **11**, 155–159.

Ryan, G. and Little, P. (1989) Problem-based learning within the School of Nursing and Health Studies at Macarthur Institute of Higher Education, in *Problem-Based Learning – The Newcastle Workshop*, (ed. B. Wallis), Faculty of Medicine University of Newcastle, NSW.

Sadler, D. (1987) Specifying and promulgating achievement standards. *Oxford Review of Education*, **13**(2), 191–209.

Sasmor, J. (1984) Contracting for clinical. *Journal of Nursing Education*, **23**(4), 171–173.

Sawer, M. and Sims, M. (1993) *A Woman's Place. Women and Politics in Australia*, Allen & Unwin, Sydney, NSW.

Schermerhorn, G. and Williams, R. (1979) An empirical comparison responsive and pre-ordinate approaches to program evaluation. *Educational Evaluation and Policy Analysis*, **1**, 55–60.

Schneider, H. (1978) *Evaluation of Nursing Competence*, Little, Brown, Boston, MA.

Schoenly, L. (1994) Teaching in the affective domain. *Journal of Nursing Education*, **25**(5), 209–212.

Schon, D. (1983) *The Reflective Practitioner: How Professionals Think in Action*, Basic Books, New York.

Schon, D. (1988) *Educating the Reflective Practitioner*, Jossey-Bass, San Francisco, CA.

Schoolcraft, V. and Delaney, C. (1982) Contract grading in clinical evaluation. *Journal of Nursing Education*, **21**, 6–14.

Schultz, B. (1989) *Communication in Small Groups*, Harper & Row, New York.

Schwirian, P. (1983) Editorial. The future is ours if. *Computers in Nursing*, **1**, 1.

Scott and Underwood (1991) Impressions of nursing. First day as a registered nurse. *The Lamp*, **48**, 5.

Sheehan, M. and Sheehan, J. (1985) The attitudes of nurse tutor students towards behavioural objectives: background and method of study. *Journal of Advanced Nursing*, **10**, 149–153.

Simon, S., Howe, L. and Kerschenbaum, H. (1978) *Values Clarification*, A & W Visual Library, New York.

Simpson, I. (1979) *From Student to Nurse*, Cambridge University Press, Cambridge.

Simpson, M. (1980) Objections to objectives. *Medical Teacher*, **2**, 229–231.

Sims, A. (1976) The critical incident technique in evaluating student nurse performance. *International Journal of Nursing Studies*, **13**, 123–131.

Singer, P. (1981) Teaching human rights, in *Teaching Human Rights*, (eds E. Kamenka and A. Tay), Australian Government Publishing Service, Canberra.

Skilbeck, M. (1984) *School Based Curriculum Development*, Harper & Row, London.

Slavinsky, A. and Diers, D. (1982) Nursing education for college graduates. *Nursing Outlook*, **30**(5), 292–297.

Smallegan, M. (1982) Teaching through groups. *Journal of Nursing Education*, **21**, 23–31.

Smith, A. and Russell, J. (1993) Critical incident technique, in *Nurse Education. A Reflective Approach*, (eds J. Reed and S. Procter), Edward Arnold, Sevenoaks, pp 119–130.

Smith, B. E. (1992) Linking theory and practice in teaching basic nursing skills. *Journal of Nursing Education*, **31**(1), 16–23.

Smith, D. and Lovat, T. (1990). *Curriculum. Action on Reflection*, Social Science Press, Wentworth Falls, NSW.

Smythe, E. (1984) *Surviving Nursing*, Addison Wesley Publishing Company, Menlo Park, CA.

Stafford, L. and Graves, C. (1978) Some problems in evaluating clinical effectiveness. *Nursing Outlook*, **26**(8), 494–497.

Stainton, M. (1983) A format for recording the clinical performance of nursing students. *Journal of Nursing Education*, **22**, 114–116.

Stecchi, J., Woltman, S., Wall-Haas, C. *et al.* (1983) Comprehensive approach to clinical evaluation: one teaching team's solution to clinical evaluation of students in multiple settings. *Journal of Nursing Education*, **22**, 38–46.

Stenhouse, L. (1975) *An Introduction to Curriculum Research and Development*, Heinemann, London.

Stevens, B. (1979) *Nursing Theory. Analysis, Application, Evaluation*, Little, Brown, Boston, MA.

Stoner, J., Collins, R. and Yetton, P. (1985) Management in Australia, Prentice Hall, Collingwood, Victoria.

Sullivan, E. and Brye, C. (1983) Nursing's future: use of the Delphi Technique for curriculum planning. *Journal of Nursing Education*, **22**, 187–189.

Swanson, E. and Dalsing, C. (1980) Independent study: a curriculum expander. *Journal of Nursing Education*, **19**, 11–15.

Sweetwood H. (1986) A framework for re-entry into nursing practice. Unpublished EdD dissertation, Teachers College, Columbia University, New York.

Taba, H. (1962) *Curriculum Development Theory and Practice*, Harcourt, Brace & World, New York.

Tanner, C. (1988) Curriculum revolution: the practice mandate, in *Curriculum Revolution: Mandate for Change*, National League for Nursing Publication No. 15-2224, National League for Nursing, New York, pp 201–216.

Tanner, C. and Lindeman, C. (1987) Research in nursing education: assumptions and priorities. *Journal of Nursing Education*, **26**(2), 50–59.

Thacker, J., Pring, R. and Evans, D. (1987) *Personal, Social and Moral Education in Changing World*, NFER Nelson, Windsor.

Thompson, I., Melia, K. and Boyd, K. (1988) *Nursing Ethics*, Churchill Livingstone, New York.

Tight, M. (ed.) (1983) *Adult Learning and Education*, Croom Helm, London .

Tinkler, D., Smith, T., Ellyard, P. and Cohen, D. (1994) *Effectiveness and Potential of Sate-of-the-Art Technologies in the Delivery of Higher Education*, Australian Government Publishing Service, Canberra.

Toffler, A. (1981) *The Third Wave*, Pan, London.

Toffler, A. and Toffler, F. (1993) *War and Anti-war. Survival at the Dawn of the 21st Century*, Little, Brown, Boston, MA.

Torres, G. and Stanton, M. (1982) *Curriculum Process in Nursing*, Prentice-Hall, Englewood Cliffs, NJ.

Turney, S., Cairns, L. Eltis, K. *et al*. (1983) *Supervisor Development Programme Role Handbook*, University of Sydney Press, Sydney, NSW.

Valiga, T. and Streubert, H. (1991) *The Nurse Educator in Academia. Strategies for Success*, Springer, New York.

Warwick, D. (1973) *Curriculum Structure and Design*, Unibooks, London.

Watts, N. (1990) *Handbook of Clinical Teaching*, Churchill Livingstone, Melbourne, Victoria.

Wealthall, S., Edwards, H. and Price, D. (1992) How to evaluate my clinical teaching. Workshop Report. *Australasian and New Zealand Association for Medical Education Bulletin*, School of Medical Education, University of New South Wales, Sydney, NSW.

Weeramantry, C. (1981) National and international systems as denigrators of human rights, in *Teaching Human Rights*, (eds E. Kamenka and A. Tay), Australian Government Publishing Service, Canberra.

Weinholtz, D and Stritter, F. (1982) How to plan an assessment of students' attitudes. *Medical Teacher*, **4**, 95–101.

White, R. and Ewan, C. (1991) *Clinical Teaching in Nursing*, Chapman & Hall, London.

White, R., Ewan, C., Hatton, N. and Lovitt, L. (1988) *Critical Incidents in Clinical Teaching. Perspectives from the Social and Behavioural Sciences: An Instructional Manual for Nurse Educators*, School of Medical Education, University of New South Wales, Sydney, NSW.

Wilson, J. (1981) *Student Learning in Higher Education*, Croom Helm, London.

Wilson, M. (1985) *Group Theory/Process for Nursing Practice*, Bowie M. D. Brady Communication Co.

Wilson-Barnett J. (1986) Ethical dilemmas in nursing. *Journal of Medical Ethics*, **12**, 123–126.

Wiseman, R. F. (1994) Role model behaviours in the clinical setting. *Journal of Nursing Education*, **33**(9), 405–410.

Woolfolk, A. (ed.) (1989) *Research Perspectives on the Graduate Preparation of Teachers*, Prentice Hall, Englewood Cliffs, NJ.

Woolley, A. (1977) The long and tortured history of clinical evaluation. *Nursing Outlook*, **25**, 308–315.

Woolridge, P. J., Skipper, J. K. and Leonard, R. C. (1968) *Behavioural Science, Social Practice and the Nursing Profession*, Press of Case Western Reserve University, Cleveland, OH.

Zimmerman, L. and Westfall, J. (1988) The development and validation of a scale measuring effective clinical teaching behaviours. *Journal of Nursing Education*, **27**(6), 274–277.

Index